BRAINSTORM

BRAINSTORM

A PERSONAL STORY

Karen Osney Brownstein

MACMILLAN PUBLISHING CO., INC.

New York

Macmillan Publishing Co., Inc.
866 Third Avenue, New York, N.Y. 10022
Collier Macmillan Canada, Ltd.

Library of Congress Cataloging in Publication Data
Brownstein, Karen Osney.
Brainstorm.
1. Brain—Tumors—Biography. 2. Brownstein,
Karen Osney. I. Title.
RC280.B7B76   362.1'969928109   79-28293
ISBN 0-02-517650-1

First Printing 1980

Printed in the United States of America

For Neill

"But there is one more thing you can learn about the body that only a nondoctor would tell you— and I hope you'll always remember this: the head bone's connected to the heart bone.
Don't let them come apart."

—ALAN ALDA
Commencement Address, Columbia University
College of Physicians and Surgeons
May 1979

ACKNOWLEDGMENTS

Brainstorm is a true story of actual events and real people. Its pages are filled with acts of skill, compassion, and endless patience by those who stood with me when the storm hit. I cannot offer thanks enough to any of them. Where names have been changed to protect the privacy of the individuals, I am no less grateful.

I began by wanting to write a funny book about a profoundly unfunny period of my life. I want to thank Howard Teichmann, a gifted writer, teacher, and generous friend, for convincing me that such a book was possible. I did not have the raw material for stand-up comedy, he wisely counseled, but neither did I have to fall into the pit of black humor.

Dr. George Perlstein of the Palo Alto Clinic has been a gentle yet unrelenting watchman, guarding the technical accuracy of the manuscript with skill, caution, and sustained good will.

Joyce Jack has managed to combine buoyant enthusiasm with insightful, close editing in behalf of *Brainstorm;* Patricia Berens, my agent, has served as a wise and bountiful touchstone from the first. Donna Lee Dowdney began by typing the manuscript and soon became one of its most responsive and intelligent critics.

I also wish to thank Ann Buyers Reedy, Mariel and Eric Donath, Janess Rosenberg, Debby Spector, Dr. Ralph J. Stiegl, Lucky Reneau, Steven Winn, Ruth Benz, Georgiana Cullen Calingo, J. P. Sanachez, and the women of *Our Stories/Ourselves.* I am grateful to them all.

Finally, were it not for the love and understanding of my family—my sons, my parents, and the man to whom this book is dedicated—there would have been no *Brainstorm.*

Karen Osney Brownstein
Palo Alto, California
June 1979

INTRODUCTION

Two years after the events in this book occurred, I sat in the office of a prominent Hollywood agent while he told me why my story about old people wouldn't sell.

"Depressing, sweetheart," he said as he drew the blinds against the California morning and lit still another cigarette with his gold Gucci lighter. "Old people are depressing. Television hates depressing. That's a fact. You want my advice? Forget old people; I can't sell 'em."

"What about film?" I said. My return flight to San Francisco didn't take off for another three hours. I had nothing to lose.

"Film isn't crazy about old people, either, you know. Black and white. The best you can hope for is black and white on a project like this. Art houses, limited distribution. No money in that, sweetheart. Trust me—old people are depressing. Go home and write one with a happy ending. You know what I mean? Everybody loves a happy ending. Besides, you're a funny writer. Go home and write funny with a happy ending and then we'll talk business."

"Would you care to hear my idea for a book about my brain tumor?"

"Jesus, kid," he said, "you're a million laughs."

BRAINSTORM

THE NEUROLOGIST WAS WEARING A MINISKIRT. You see, smarty-pants! I scolded myself. You see what happens when you finally act on your high-minded feminist principles and actually go to a woman doctor. What happens is that you wind up in the competent hands of Little Bo Peep, M.D.

Bo Peep, whose name was Melinda Marks, watered all of the plants in her Wedgwood-blue office at the Neurological Institute of Columbia Presbyterian Medical Center before acknowledging me. I felt invisible.

"What makes you think you need a neurologist?" she finally asked. She was climbing on and off chairs to reach hanging plants.

I don't, is what I wanted to say to her. I don't and so good-bye, good luck, Godspeed. And by the way, honey, you've got great legs! So you just stick to your guns. Who cares if no one with any style has been caught dead in a miniskirt for the last ten years. You just stick with it, lady, and I'll be running along now.

Exit new patient.

In fact, I said none of this and begrudgingly told the truth.

"I get headaches."

"What kind of headaches?" she asked while slipping on a fresh, white lab coat that nearly reached her ankles. Sitting behind her mahogany desk, she seemed so much more substantial that I began to take this appointment more seriously.

"Frequent headaches," I said, admiring my careful word choice. "Frequent, intense headaches." There now. That ought to separate me from the rest of the thirtyish female hypochondriacs, I thought happily.

"Mm hmm," was Melinda's nonresponse. I was beginning to wish she had more plants to water when a nervous young woman came in and silently took a chair behind the doctor.

his is Betsy, my resident," said Melinda Marks. Sweet-faced
nodded a head of blond curls at me and smiled shyly. Bo
heep.

This is Karen Brownstein, Betsy. She's here because she gets
headaches." This time Betsy nodded with clear-eyed concentration.
Her mentor was speaking, and if Melinda Marks was saying Karen
gets headaches, well, then, no doubt about it, Karen gets headaches.
In fact, she was getting one now.

"How long have you been getting them?" Melinda was asking.
That was a tougher question than it sounded. In fact, it was hard to
remember when I hadn't had some kind of headaches. Maybe I ought
to tell it all. Yes. What the hell, I was going to leave with the same
Valium prescription whether I enjoyed this visit or not. Why not be
honest? In ten days I'd be moving to California with my husband
and two young sons, no matter what. And once settled in sunny
Palo Alto I would certainly get over these headaches, which were
surely caused by the tension born of a cross-country move. Yes. I'd
tell it all. It beat packing moving boxes.

"How long? Well, for the last three years I've been seeing an ear-
nose-and-throat man for sinus headaches. He gives me those terrific
little needles in the nose."

"Needles in the *what?*" Melinda and Betsy said in unison.

"Nose. It's a local treatment that uses some kind of oil-based
steroids. I began getting the injections when I was pregnant three
years ago and didn't want to be swallowing pills. I know it sounds
barbaric, but actually it's only uncomfortable. And the shots really
do work. Every three to five months I'd whip up here to Dr. Miles,
lay my head back, and he'd fire away—twice. One for each—"

"*Barry* Miles?" Melinda interrupted. "Barry's a friend of mine.
We have coffee together every morning. Funny he's never mentioned this treatment."

"Well, he ought to. It's the most magically effective medical treatment I've ever had. Two zaps and the headaches are gone. Actually
a three-visit series, but what's the difference? That they work is
the point. Or at least they did, until the last round."

"What happened then?"

"I don't know. But the magic was somehow gone. This time there
was no instant cure and I still had headaches. Lots of them. In fact, a
few weeks ago, when my husband was in California on a business
trip, a headache woke me up. From a sound sleep. Ordinarily it
takes a very sexy man or a very sick child to wake me in the middle
of the night." Melinda and Betsy exchanged a look I could not read.

4

"Is that when you called Mike?" Melinda asked.

Michael Margolin is a good friend who happens to be a fine neurologist. When he and his wife Dorrie chose to move to Moorestown, New Jersey, where Mike set up practice, it left a sad space in our lives. It was Mike who'd sent me to Melinda Marks, but only when the first two doctors he'd recommended were unable to see me. That she was his third choice gave me pause; but my concern was mitigated when I learned that *she* could not fit me in for nearly two weeks.

The crazy dynamics of big city medicine: if you want to see the "big guns," chances are you'll either be dead or cured before your appointment rolls around. Perhaps that's how famous doctors earn their reputations for dramatic cures—they're consistently unavailable for small ills. A doctor once defended this practice to me by describing it as "maximum efficiency talent distribution."

Anyway, that was not when I had called Mike.

"I called him about three weeks ago when I had a nightmare." Again they exchanged meaningful looks. "I dreamt I had a brain tumor."

This time Betsy nodded so hard I feared her head might roll straight into her lap.

"What did Mike say?" Melinda asked.

"Oh, that he doubted I had anything quite so exotic. And that, while he wasn't exactly alarmed, he thought that headache pain strong enough to wake me should be investigated."

"How often did it wake you?"

"Once. No . . . twice. Just twice."

She drew a clean sheet of paper from the top drawer of her beautiful desk and made a notation.

"Tell me about the headaches," she said.

"What do you want to know?"

"Oh, you know," she answered. "Where does it hurt? How often? How long does the pain last? Like that. Tell me about it."

I was beginning to like her style. Loose, easy, none of that "when did you have your tonsils out—how old are you—how many children" nonsense. Just "tell me about it."

So I told her how I'd had the headaches for months. How each headache lasted for only a few moments—but while they lasted, the flashes of pain behind my eyes were brutal. Over time the intervals between headaches had grown shorter, and the pain more acute. I'd even begun to substitute television for reading because it was a more effective tranquilizer, a quicker escape from the pain

5

that reading seemed to intensify. Of course I took the opportunity to take a few potshots at current TV fare. It's almost impossible for old English majors to step forward and admit to being closet TV freaks. But certainly in this instance, where it was being used as a substitute for pain-killers, it was acceptable, I said.

"Does the pain interfere with your life?"

"Not really." I had a sudden recollection of the day I was to take my three-year-old son, Todd, to the Bronx Zoo with several of his playmates. I sat on the kitchen floor and cried, trying to explain to him that we couldn't go because Mommy had a hurt in her head. But that was really the only time.

"Well, actually, just a few cancelled appointments. Nothing major," I said lightly.

"Do you work?" she wanted to know. I told her I was an on-again, off-again freelance writer.

"What do you write?" Perhaps because so few people had asked that lately, or because when Mike was naming neurologists he had referred to the males as Dr. Thus-and-Such and to her as simply "Melinda Marks," I told her the truth.

"I write about feminist comedy."

"No kidding! Tell me about it." Again, "tell me about it." I really began to enjoy her.

"Well, it's comedy about women's bodies. Kind of a female Lenny Bruce approach." She seemed to perk up at that reply.

"You mean you write about tits and ass?" She was actually wide-eyed now.

"That's right. And gynecologists and dressing gowns and belt-less sanitary napkins. Not insulting to women, though. Not like Joan Rivers, say, or Phyllis Diller and her mini-bra. My humor is, pardon the expression, more supportive of women."

"Can you sell that sort of thing?" Betsy asked softly.

"Not very easily," I admitted. I liked this. I liked Betsy and I liked Melinda and I liked talking about my writing. And I certainly liked it better than talking about my headaches. But Melinda had had enough fun for a Wednesday morning. She told me to go into the adjacent examining room and get undressed—down to my underpants. My underpants?

It must have been all that talk about women's bodies, I thought as I pulled my pink T-shirt over my head. Why else would I have to strip for headaches? No, it must be that Dr. Marks didn't get all that many cracks at pornographers—in the flesh.

6

To the casual observer, a complete neurological examination must look a lot like "show time at the funny farm."

"Close your eyes. Now touch your nose with the third finger of your left hand. Good. Now the right hand . . . that's fine. Now jump off the table and, without watching your feet, walk heel-to-toe across the room in a straight line. No, you may not open your eyes." As if the tasks were not ridiculous enough, there is the added embarrassment of hearing the commands rendered with perfect sobriety. This is not, after all, a simple game of "Simon Says." No one laughs if you forget to say "Mother, may I?"

If walking the straight line doesn't knock you out of the game, you proceed immediately to the push-and-shove segment of the examination. The technique is quite simple: the doctor holds up his finger, or better still his whole hand, and your job as patient is to push it down. Force and counterforce. Neuromuscular response. All very basic. Except that some folks really get into these little maneuvers, patients and doctors alike.

Take it from me. If Melinda Marks ever gives up medicine, she has a very promising career as a lady wrestler.

When all the silly stuff is over, the small bag of tricks gets opened. The small black bag that contains the neurologist's tools of the trade is recognizable anywhere—neonatologists notwithstanding, no doctor's bag is smaller.

Out of it comes the hook or tickler to check reflexes on the soles of your feet. Splendid. Also the delicate rubber-edged hammer that's used for tapping your knees and other places.

These are fairly universal tools. But a small space in the bag is given over to the individual practitioner's creativity. For example, in order to test the most subtle variances in response, a Q-tip may be drawn across your (closed) eyelids. The doctor will ask if there is any difference in the way you perceive the touch with the left or right eye. For this delicate exercise, Melinda Marks carried a pigeon feather. Creative, no?

And yet with all the games and paraphernalia, Melinda was coming up dry on the question of my headaches. Until she looked at my eyes.

Using an opthalmoscope, the round-headed instrument that gives the physician a window to the brain, Melinda stared for long moments into my eyes. She stepped back silently. The smart-assed banter between two bright, hip women was gone.

"C'mere Betsy. Take a look at her eyes." So Betsy, with none of the timidity that had marked her earlier participation, came and held her face inches from mine and looked. And learned.

"There's something funny in her eyes," Melinda said from a few paces back. "See it?" Betsy nodded. She could see it.

What? "What!" I wanted to say to both of them. No, *shout* at both of them. But I said nothing while Melinda had another look.

"Put on your clothes and come into the office," she said in a voice so toneless it chilled my heart.

For the first of what were to be many such times, I found a way to block the fear that was leaping through my body. I would concentrate on the task: all of my thoughts turned to the pink T-shirt and pants that lay on the chair. The birds on the T-shirt were hummingbirds. Funny, I'd never noticed that. The pants were really too long when worn with these shoes. Make a note of that. At the small mirror hanging on the examining room wall, I smoothed my long dark hair, carefully avoiding my own eyes.

Melinda and Betsy were each scribbling notes when I walked into the office. No one had to tell me to sit down. When at last Melinda spoke, no words were wasted.

"There's something in your head that shouldn't be there," she said.

"Like what?" I asked. "You mean, like a tumor?"

"Yes, I think so. Probably. We'll need to do some tests, of course, but—"

"Wait a minute. Are you telling me I have a brain tumor? That I may die soon?"

"Yes, I think that's quite possible, but. . . ."

Whatever she said next was lost on me. In fairness to her, there may have been a long string of qualifiers, but I heard none then and I can remember none now. Only the words "Yes, I think that's quite possible" came through. No softness, no kindness. No modifiers. Nothing to soften the blow.

When at last I could speak, I asked to call my husband, who was on a business trip in California. That was premature, Melinda counseled. Why not wait until after the test results began coming in? But I knew better.

Eighteen months earlier, Neill had been in California on a similar trip when I had admitted myself for emergency abdominal surgery

8

into a New York hospital. By the time he got off the plane I was out of surgery, out of the recovery room, and out of courage. There was no way I'd let that happen this time. If Melinda disapproved, tough! I wanted him with me, and as fast as United Airlines could deliver him. While I couldn't think clearly enough to calculate the East to West Coast time difference and the flight time, I knew that, at best, it would be the middle of the night before he could be home. I was going to call him, no matter what she said.

With no graciousness whatever, Melinda allowed me to make the call from her office while she turned her back to me and used another line to set up a schedule of tests for that afternoon.

While Neill kept saying it couldn't be true, Melinda kept making the arrangements that would prove it was or wasn't.

In short order she was ushering me out of her Wedgwood-blue jungle. All business, she handed me two hospital orders and gave me instructions for finding my way through the labyrinth of underground tunnels that would bring me to my first destination—skull X-rays.

An hour before we'd been pals, she and I—laughing at my stories, joyfully empathizing with each other's achievements.

"It would help, Dr. Marks," I said at her office doorway, "if you could just hold my hand for a minute or two."

"I can't," she answered matter-of-factly. "But Betsy will." And Betsy, sweet-faced, bowled-over Betsy did. All the way to Radiology where the pictures showed nothing and then all the way to the electroencephalogram.

As I lay on the narrow table, wires attached to my head as though I were some space-age Medusa, Betsy whispered that she had to leave. If I didn't kiss her pale hand, I should have.

NEUROLOGICAL INSTITUTE SITS LIKE A GRAY, MEDIEVAL FORTRESS at the northern tip of Manhattan. Across Fort Washington Avenue are the major buildings of Columbia Presbyterian Medical Center; behind is the Hudson River.

The cognoscenti call this building "Neuro." Until the recent construction of the medical library just north of it, Neuro's closest institutional neighbor was Psychiatric Institute. That seemed appropriate to me.

I could see this institutional panorama from a window in Melinda Marks's office. This was to be the rendevous point following the electroencephalogram. I was trying to brush from my hair the thick gluey substance used to attach the wires when she came striding in, her lab coat flapping.

"Nothing. Perfect. Clean as a whistle," she announced without a trace of feeling.

Ha, ha, Bo Peep! Lost your sheep? Jumped the gun a little, didn't you? Scared the hell out of me for nothing? I can take the Valium and run.

"The CAT scan will tell it all," she said cooly. "C'mon. Let's go down there and let the old CAT have a look at you."

"The what?"

"The CAT brain scan. Stands for *computerized axial tomography*. Greatest thing since the X-ray."

In the elevator I bombarded her with questions. How could a tumor be present in my brain if the X-rays and the EEG showed nothing? How could a healthy young woman just coming into her goddam prime have a brain tumor and not know it? How?

"Look," she explained as she signed me in for the CAT scan, "you've had two good tests. But when I looked into your eyes this morning, I saw more papilledema than I'd ever seen in a patient.

Well, that's not exactly true," she amended. "In a patient who wasn't comatose."

"More what?" I repeated. "Papille . . . what?"

"*Papilledema*," she pronounced. "It means that when I look into your eyes I can see swelling around the optic nerve. It's engorged, distended. There's too much pressure in your head. Something's in there, causing all that pressure. The scan can take thin, cross-sectional pictures of your brain and tell us what that something is." I was back in her flock.

"Let me go see if we can't get you in there now," she said. While we walked down the silent corridor, passing the inner sanctums of Columbia's leading lights in radiology, Melinda explained the CAT scan to me in layperson's terms. This scan, she told me, is a fantastic diagnostic tool that has revolutionized the practice of neurology. It is also a very costly device and in short supply.

"Every flake who gets a headache wants a crack at it," she said. There would almost certainly be a wait before my turn. Did I want to get a cup of coffee? I tried hard to believe that I would have had to wait even if my doctor were a man, and agreed to meet her in another hour.

This was my "free time." Time in which to contemplate the cataclysmic storm of events that had brought me to the basement floor of a building I'd heard Mike call "the house of hope and horrors."

Time for praying that I was nothing more than a flake who gets headaches.

Time to call my wonderful friend Edye and ask her to take care of my children. She listened in silence as I recounted the morning's events. Not for nothing was Edye a graduate fellow in psychology. Even her silence was comforting.

"I love you," she said simply when I had finished. "When shall I tell Adam and Todd you'll be home?"

"Not for miles," I sighed. And for the first time that day, I cried.

When I was twelve I read movie magazines. About that time Joan Crawford was widowed and I remembered an interview in which she was asked how she managed to seem so charming even as she was grieving.

"I cry on my own time," had been her answer. This was my own time.

I wrote a love letter to Neill. With any luck at all he'd be on a plane by now, but I needed to share these moments with him.

And I went for a walk in the June sunlight. Around and around that gray maze of hospital buildings I marched, chanting little staccato prayers:

> Test one is good.
> Test two is good.
> Now please, God,
> Make it three.

When it was time to go back for the scan, I had marched and chanted my way into solitary numbness. I passed Billy Di Mauro without recognizing him.

"Karen?" he said with the lilting Italian accent he'd brought with him when he came to New York to do research at Neuro and become my Riverdale high-rise neighbor in the process.

"Oh, my God, Billy," I cried. "You'll never believe it!"

Billy held my hand as we walked back into the gray building. I was not going to be alone with my nightmare after all. I had a friend at Neuro—a warm, sensitive, and, perhaps most important, knowledgeable friend.

A three-year-old girl had fallen or been pushed from a five-story tenement window. Hers was the brain "scanned" in Room B2 before mine. Her shrieks filled the hallway. Was it terror that made the child wail, I wondered, or pain? Both, I decided sadly.

"Don't let that get to you," Melinda said abruptly. "At least she's conscious. I'll meet you down here when you're through."

"Me too," Billy said and he hugged me.

I was alone again. Even the lead door could not keep the child's cries from reaching me. Time to tune out again. The small, deserted waiting area had the obligatory out-of-date magazines; I would read old *Sports Illustrated*s while I waited for my turn.

The door of Room B2 opened and a chubby, smiling young man came through it. He watched me silently until I could no longer ignore him. When I looked up he was grinning.

"You waiting for a brain scan?" he asked cheerfully.

"Yes."

"Ever had one before?"

"No."

"You're going to love it."

My God, I thought, the hospital planner who'd put this place so close to Psychiatric Institute was nobody's fool.

"No, really," he went on. "This is my fourth. And if you can get into it, a CAT scan is really a trip. I mean, it doesn't hurt or anything. And that waterbag. Well, I mean, it's so relaxing I actually fell asleep in there today."

"What's your name?"

"John. John Ubeleski. What's yours?" I told him. I told him all about me. My headaches, my husband, my children, my moving to California. By the time I had finished telling him, the child was quiet.

"Don't be afraid," he said. "That thing saved my life." He was halfway down the hall when he turned around and came back.

"Hey, listen," he said shyly. "Would you do me a favor when you get to California?"

"Sure," I said. I expected it would be a phone call to a maiden aunt.

"Plant a flower for me."

Although it's not marked as such, there's a good chunk of my backyard known as the John Ubeleski Gardens.

———————————
———————————
———————————

"You catch more flies with sugar than you do with vinegar," my English grandmother had instructed me. It was a maxim that had not yet failed. It had worked as I was growing up in Chicago and worked when I was a student in New York. A classmate of mine, a native New Yorker, once said she'd never met anyone who used "please" and "thank you" with so much success. "I can't believe it!" she exclaimed after a shopping trip to Bloomingdale's. "You even say it to *salesclerks*. Nobody says it to salesclerks!" Neuro is only one hundred and seven blocks uptown from Bloomingdale's. It couldn't hurt, I thought.

"May I please have something to support my shoulders?" I asked after my head had been fitted into the machine that would "tell it all." The rest of me lay flat on a cushioned table.

"Sure," said the smiling technician. "We'll get you a rubber pillow for your neck." Chalk up another one for Grandma.

A CAT scan was not exactly the day in the country John Ubeleski had promised. First of all, there was the strange way machine and patient were made to come together. Remember the old steam boxes that were a standard prop in every comedy routine about fat? Before we were all so tuned into nutrition and exercise, even before

13

Weight Watchers, there was a box that was meant to steam away pounds. You sat in it with your head sticking out. With a brain scan, it's just the opposite: your head goes in and your body sticks out.

Just as the technician was closing the lead door—a move that signified the beginning of the test—I began to laugh, aloud. He came back in.

"Is anything wrong, Karen?" he asked kindly.

"No," I said, trying not to giggle. "It's just . . . well, do you remember that old joke—it's a fourth-grade joke, I think—that began, 'Do you wanna lose ten pounds of ugly fat?' "

"No, I don't remember it. What's the punch line?"

"Cut off your head!" I trilled. He chuckled politely and tightened my chin strap. My laughing had loosened it.

For the next hour and a half I couldn't think of any more fourth-grade jokes. All I seemed able to think about was escape. Going home. Getting away. Let me go plant my flowers in California.

Billy was waiting for me when the door to B2 opened. He looked terrible.

"We've already got the pictures," Melinda Marks said, fingering a Billie Jean King cover of *Sports Illustrated*. "There's a ton of pressure on your brain."

"From what?" I asked. My knees were giving way. Billy brought a chair while Melinda explained.

"The cerebrospinal fluid in your head is building up, not circulating the way it's supposed to." Somehow that didn't sound so awful to me.

"Then that's what's giving me the headaches, not a tumor?" I asked, nearly hopeful.

"I didn't say that," she said. "There's so much fluid in those pictures it's impossible to see what's blocking its passage." Billy put his hand on mine.

"And what do you do about that?" I asked her.

"I don't do anything. A neurosurgeon does it." I looked desperately at Billy.

"An operation? On my brain?" Billy was looking at his lap.

"Yes. And the sooner the better," Melinda said. "Probably tomorrow, Friday at the latest. I've already notified the O.R."

"She means the operating room," Billy said gently, breaking his silence. "It's really not such a bad operation. Karen," he said in slow and perfect English, "you must have it."

A fist had grown in my throat.

14

"I want to go home," I said, rising with difficulty. "I want to go home and come back tomorrow. Please, Dr. Marks."

She raised her eyebrows at Billy. Could I be trusted?

"For God's sake, lady! I'm not going to ditch you. I just want to go home and see my children and sleep with my husband in my own bed and I'll come back here first thing in the morning! Please!"

She said yes and Billy drove me home.

Really, Karen, neurosurgically speaking, it's a small operation," Billy said as we drove along the Henry Hudson Parkway. The sun was low on the river beside us.

"A small operation on my brain."

"Yes, a small tube is inserted to drain the fluid." He turned off onto the Riverdale exit and was quiet. As we pulled into the driveway of our high-rise building just a few miles up the river from the hospital, I was stunned. The building, the flowers bordering the circular driveway—everything looked just the same as when I'd left that morning. My world had caved in while everything else had stayed the same. How was that possible?

Billy rode the elevator up to the fourteenth floor with me and pressed the "open door" button, prolonging his departure.

"Do you want me to stay?" he asked kindly.

"No, I'll be all right, Billy. Honestly. You've already done more than I can ever thank you for. But Billy . . . there's just one thing. . . . Do you think I should have another opinion?"

His face tighened. "I saw the films," he said. "You must have the operation right away. Should I stay?"

"No," I whispered. "I'll be fine."

I walked into my apartment, my head bursting with pain, and cried until I thought the pain would crack my head the way a nutcracker splits a walnut. Wouldn't *that* save the neurosurgeon a lot of time, I thought while I ran cold water over my face. I was full of bizarre fantasies. There was no way I was prepared to face my three- and six-year-old sons in this condition.

"Edye," I said into the telephone, "I'm home, but I'm not ready yet—not myself. Can you keep them another hour? I need to get myself together." Of course. Wonderful Edye . . . wonderful Billy

16

. . . wonderful husband . . . wonderful kids . . . wonderful life, I thought as I reached for the aspirin bottle on the kitchen counter.

"Grim Reaper," I said aloud. "You got some rotten timing!" And that's how I began to get myself together. Talking to myself.

"All right," I said to the breakfast dishes that were still in the sink, "let's think this whole thing through. We're in big trouble here. No doubt about it. Now—do we want to tough it out or call in the reserves?" Funny thing about those dishes: they answered me. They didn't actually speak; I wasn't *that* far gone. But what they did do was multiply right before my eyes. Where there had been two cereal bowls, there were now four; one juice glass was two. Forks were reproducing themselves in the sink.

"Ever see double?" Melinda Marks had asked me in her office.

"No." Not until this moment. Call in the reserves! At once!

I made three phone calls. My parents. My friend Jack, who happened to be a football player turned rabbi, and Michael Margolin.

"Oh, shit! No!" Mike said when I'd told him. "Not you!"

"Why not me?"

"I just never thought it could happen to someone I cared about," he said. "Someone so healthy. So young. No other symptoms, right? Just the headaches, isn't that what you said?"

"That's what I said. That's all there were. Mike? What are they going to do to me?"

"A shunt," Mike said. "They'll put in a shunt to relieve the pressure. Dammit, I wish I were there!"

"You already are," I said. "If it weren't for you, I'd be packing moving boxes right now, preparing for life in a fool's paradise. According to Melinda Marks, calling you was the first step in saving my own life." I could hear him sigh.

"This whaddayacallit, Mike, this *shunt*? Is it really not such a big deal?" He laughed such a good-natured long-distance laugh that he might have been standing in the kitchen beside me.

"Listen, Kare, a shunt is bread-and-butter neurosurgery. Compared to most of the procedures those guys do on brains, this one is a piece of cake. They even let me have a go at it once, so you know it can't be a biggie."

The call to my parents in Florida was harder, but it could not be postponed. Not if I wanted to see them before my bread-and-butter surgery. I rehearsed the line until I could say it without my voice cracking: "Please try not to be alarmed, but come."

My rational mother cried while my stoic father rationalized.

Weren't there going to be more tests? Hmm? Hadn't I just said there were going to be more tests before the surgery? Well, maybe those tests would come up winners. Maybe I wouldn't need the operation after all.

"Daddy," I said as calmly as I could, "whatever the tests show, it isn't going to be good. That much is clear. Now tell Mother to stop crying and start packing."

By eight-thirty my children were asleep. I'd managed an astonishingly successful performance of *The Plucky Mommy* while Edye stood in the wings in case I became so distraught that I blew it. I pulled it off, though—stories, lullabies, the whole show.

"C'mon," I told Edye. "Come keep me company while I do something with this face. I've got guests arriving in a little while."

So Edye sat on the toilet seat while Revlon and I collaborated. Apart from the gunk that still stuck stubbornly to my hair, I looked like the hostess. Of course the fact that the hostess couldn't bear to be alone with her own reflection wasn't lost on Edye.

"Can you stand a little friendly advice?" Edye asked as we stood in the kitchen while I filled an ice bucket.

"I think so," I said. "What is it?"

"Get rid of the hummingbirds. They're simply not for evening, my dear."

I went to the bedroom and changed. The let's-keep-Karen's-spirits-up party deserved better.

Well, possibly not, I thought by the time the party should have been in full swing. Some swing—my friends were sitting around with faces down to my high-pile carpeting, while I vainly attempted to make them feel better.

"Look at it this way," I said to the gathering of my dear friends. "If it hadn't been for that spooky dream, I would have moved blissfully off to California next week and died among perfect strangers. This way I have you!" Silence. Not even a snicker. No doubt abut it, I was bombing in my own living room. I tried another tack.

"Listen," I said. "You all know my mother." My blond, blue-eyed Jewish mother doesn't have a stereotypical bone in her body; but I was desperate enough to make her the butt of a Jewish-mother joke worthy of Sam Levenson.

"Now, when she walks in here, the first thing she's going to ask is: 'Have you eaten anything?' I want you to watch carefully and then sign pledge cards." While they watched I slowly peeled a banana and even more slowly ate it.

"When she gets here, I want you to head her off at the pass." My friend Jeff stood up and headed for the door.

"I can't handle this," he said simply. "Tell my wife I'm walking home."

I was losing them fast. While I poured yet another bottle of wine, Jack came into the kitchen and put his arms around me. How he'd ever found his way from the Texas defensive line to the rabbinate was no small miracle in itself.

"How you doin', babe?" he asked in a rich Houston drawl.

"Fine. Oh, Jack! Rotten. Remember Don Meredith after the Dallas Cowboys lost the Superbowl in 1970?"

"Yeah," he said still gripping me in a bear hug.

"Well, the next night he went on the Johnny Carson show and old John asked him what he thought had gone wrong. And Meredith, well, he wiped away a tear and said, looking straight at the camera, 'Ah played harrible! Ah jus' played harrible.' Well that's how I feel, Jack. Just like Meredith. I've let everybody down."

"Now hold on a minute, honey . . ." Jack began.

"No. No! Dammit, Jack, I don't want to die now! I don't want to leave Neill and Adam and Todd and you and my writing and my. . . ." I couldn't get the rest out for a long time. "How do I make God understand that? How do I ask Him to stop all this right now? To make it not be a brain tumor? To make it be something I can deal with? How?"

"You don't, babe," Jack said slowly. "You don't pray that it be this or that. You don't go makin' deals with God. What you can pray for is the strength and the understanding to face whatever it is that comes next. That's a prayer God can answer for you." That's a prayer worth passing along, I came to realize.

By the time my parents rang the doorbell it was 1 A.M. Nobody had left since Jeff. My mother sobbed and rocked me in her arms. It made me cry for my own sleeping babies. My father, whom I was forever criticizing for his tight-lipped macho, stood in the hallway and made Mother and me look like amateurs.

When there were no tears left, we walked through the foyer into the suddenly hushed living room. My mother took one look at the fruit bowl and delivered the line that finally got my party rolling.

19

For a while there it was nearly fun. You can't throw Texans and New Yorkers into the same pot and not have something cooking. I could stop trying so hard.

When at last I heard Neill's key in the door I jumped up and ran to meet him. White-faced and haggard, he looked like a man who'd wandered into the wrong apartment. Whatever he'd expected as he flew home, it was not this—not a party.

The place cleared out in no time. It was three o'clock in the morning, and I was due at the hospital by eight.

———————————
———————————
———————————

A short lesson in sex role stereotypes: when Neill graduated from high school, his senior class awarded him the coveted distinction of Most Masculine. It was 1962. In those days "most masculine" translated as captain of the football team, hairy chest, and successful with virgins.

The very same senior class chose me as the Girl Most Likely to Succeed, meaning big brain, big mouth, and as my father so indelicately phrased it, smart-assed broad. My best friend Barbara had a nicer way with words. "Achievement-oriented," she announced to me after a semester of Psych I. "That's what you are."

When I got to Barnard, the poorest but proudest of the elite eastern women's colleges, the place was lousy with big brains. The message there was not subtle but a clarion call: "You are the women who will (choose one) run for president, cure cancer, teach at Harvard Law School. Now get out there girls, and sic 'em!" I loved it, every wonderful pressure-packed minute of it. The women's movement was just around the corner and I knew I was in the right place at the right time.

While I gloried in the heady teachings of Barnard faculty Kate Millett and Catherine Stimpson, Neill was across the street at Columbia with Lionel Trilling, Moses Hadas, and Peter Kennen. He was still playing football, but anyone who's ever followed the Ivy League can tell you what an exercise in humility that must have been.

When we married in 1966, there were still some folks back home in Chicago who thought that the linking of the "most masculine" with the "girl most likely to succeed" meant I'd fulfilled my manifest destiny, but neither Neill nor I was among them.

We loved each other with passion, pride, and humility. And we

20

worked at it. All that achievement orientation, his and mine, found its way into our union. There was no competition; only this heady, shared ego strength. Each of us thought the other pretty hot stuff; but together? Together we were unshakable.

Tonight we trembled in each other's arms.

"We'll make it," Neill whispered in the dawn light. Our bodies were wet with love and tears.

"We?"

"Damn betcha!"

WE WERE CATAPULTED INTO WAKEFULNESS BY THE RAUCOUS SOUND OF THE ROLLING STONES. The clock radio went off at six-thirty, an absurdly unnecessary alarm. I looked closely at Neill; he had the wide-awake stare of the shell-shocked. As I moved toward him, he closed his eyes.

"I'll go make coffee," I whispered. The apartment was ominously still as I opened the bedroom door; it too seemed to be waiting. Moving boxes stood everywhere, wall-to-wall reminders that the future had been put on "hold."

In the boys' room, Adam slept tight against the naked wall, and Todd murmured in his crib. The Babar posters, the Playschool toys, the brightly covered books were all packed away in boxes neatly labeled "Todd's Books," "Adam's Books," "Todd's Toys," "Adam's Toys." In California they'd each have a room of their own. It had taken me a full weekend to do the sorting, all the while knowing I was probably creating more problems than order.

I walked down the hall, through the sunny yellow living room, to the far end of the apartment where the library-den had been hastily converted into a guest room for my parents. Their door was closed. I knocked softly.

"We're up," my mother said. "Open the door."

This room seemed to me the saddest of all. In it was every box that didn't actually know where it was going. Four cartons carefully marked "Karen's Miscellaneous—DO NOT TOUCH" reached almost to the ceiling. In them were every diary I had kept since the sixth grade, my academic awards, degrees, love letters, blue-books from college final exams, the first drafts of every poem or short story or play I'd ever written, letters and cards and port-

22

folios—thick brown envelopes that held my vague hopes of linking my past careers with the suddenly unreal future.

Uttering the cant of the career mother in conflict, I'd told myself "when the children are older" as I had sifted through the materials. I'd spent three years as a high school English teacher. Somewhere in one huge, expandable envelope were whole units on *King Lear*, *Great Expectations*, *One Flew Over the Cuckoo's Nest*, and a two-inch stack of earnestly corrected but never returned senior themes. When I left teaching I told those seniors that while I was doing such an outstanding job of teaching Thoreau's *Walden* (which all but a few of them had hated), I'd convinced myself that the beat of *my* drummer could not be heard in the halls of Niles Township High School East. It was time to follow it elsewhere.

The elsewhere was contained in the second oversize envelope standing against the wall. "Advertising" said the masking tape pasted across it. Inside were whole ad campaigns for Chicago's leading yogurt company and a potpourri of things written in behalf of the McGovern-for-president campaign.

It was all here in the boxes. Someday I'd pull it all out and come to terms with being a full-time working mother. Someday.

"How you doing, Bop?" my father said from under his blanket. He hadn't called me that in years, not since I was a little girl. It wasn't a big jump from Bop to smart-assed broad with my father. No small part of my assertiveness and self-confidence was due to a father who treated me, guided me, and advised me no differently than he did my brother.

My father's philosophy was tripartite: (1) God hates cowards; (2) God helps those who help themselves; (3) You can't hit the pitches unless you swing at them.

Nobody was swinging at pitches this morning. This morning I was Bop again.

"Do you want me to make breakfast?" my mother mumbled against the pillows. Like Neill, she couldn't open her eyes to me.

"No, that's all right. Nobody's up yet. I'll make coffee and I'll call you when it's ready." Other times she'd have argued with me. Other times.

Other times she had come to help me get settled in a new city, to help me when my babies were born. Other times. Other times we'd laugh and tease each other and trade eye-shadow and secrets. Not this time, though—not now.

23

"All right, sweetheart, you make the coffee." I could see her face now, the beautiful face that for years had been mistaken for my sister's. Overnight she had aged twenty years. My lovely mother looked like she'd just gone five rounds with Melinda Marks, lady wrestler.

As I walked back through the living room, bare now of all the paintings and plants and small treasures that had made this our home for six years, I thought how much more it seemed like a warehouse than a place where a family lived.

Through the floor-to-ceiling windows that stretched the length of the room I could see the first rays of the June sun gently touching the Hudson River. The flame-red geraniums, tended with city gardener dedication through three summers, shone in the window boxes we'd hung along the terrace railing. These were all that was left of the small jungle I'd worked so hard to maintain in New York. With the arrogance of unlimited fertility, the state of California did not allow plants grown elsewhere to cross its borders, so I'd given my house plants away in a gesture that revealed exactly where my friends stood with me.

The prize palm, the one that would have made the managers of the Palm Court at the Plaza weep, went to Lucky, the soft-spoken Honduran woman who had been my household helper, friend, and New-York-grandmother-in-residence to my children for six years. And although she had the worst exposures for growing things, Edye got the best of the rest. The others were divided with an even hand among the women who had shared with me the unique and sometimes bizarre intimacy of our young mothering years.

Only the geraniums were left. They were to be a gift to the new tenants of apartment 14E. The new tenants! My God, I had not thought of it until now! In ten days the lease was theirs. We'd have no place to live! I'd be recovering from brain surgery and we'd be homeless. I raced to the bedroom, pain whipping through my head like the blades of a blender.

"Neill!" I whispered hysterically. "Wake up! What about the movers? The lease! Where will we live?" I was trembling.

"It's all on my list," Neill said softly. "The movers, the rental agent, the agent in California, the kid's day-camps in Palo Alto. It's all on my list. I'll handle it. Don't even think about things like that. Just trust me."

"Oh, my poor darling," I sobbed, leaning over him. "It's all on your head now, isn't it? I'm so sorry. I'm so damn sorry." Ah played harrible. I was letting everybody down. What I had told Jack was true.

Neill raised his head to look at the clock. I could hear the children waking up.

"You start packing," he said, rising and putting on his blue terry cloth robe. "I'll go tell the kids that their mother won't be home for a while." He closed the door to our room behind him.

Their mother. I stood in front of the bathroom mirror and let it all hit me. I might not be their mother forever. I might be dead very soon. Someone else might be their mother. A stranger might be their mother.

For nearly twenty-four hours I'd held a steel curtain between me and my children. With one horrible scream I smashed right through it.

"No! . . . No!" I screamed at the mirror. A scream so fierce it shot bolt after bolt of crackling pain through my skull.

"It has to be me," I sobbed. "Nobody else . . . they're mine. Oh, God, don't take me away from them. They're mine!"

Adam. Adam was six. If I died now he'd be old enough to remember me. Would he? Would he remember? Would he remember the countless hours of swings and slides and songs we made up together? Where could a stranger find a space between me and the sweet intensity of that child? How could she know what to say to a boy who at five had come to me with his first original story and said to me, "We're alike, Mommy, you and me. We both can make up books."

"Oh, Adam," I cried in the empty bathroom. "My darling black-eyed lamb! Please! Please remember! Tell Todd too."

Todd would not remember. He was two and a half—hovering on the border of conscious memory. All of the sunlit fall afternoons I sat nursing him and crooning melodies I'd made up just for him would be as nothing. Would the stranger be able to see past the dimples and the thick dark lashes to the devilish gleam in my baby's knowing eyes?

"He's funny, stranger," I whispered. "He's got the best damn sense of humor you're ever going to know. Don't confuse it with plain mischievousness. He's special! He's mine."

There was a soft, tentative knock on the bathroom door.

"Mommy?" It was Adam. "Grandma's going to take us down to Edye's house. We just wanna say good-bye before Daddy drives you to the hospital."

25

"I'm coming out, honey. Just a minute." There was neither time nor water enough to rinse away the tormented face in the mirror. I opened the door and knelt to him.

"Were you crying, Mom?" Adam asked while Todd stood silently behind him. There was no more steel curtain. I pulled them both to me and wept.

"Why are you crying?" Adam asked as he patted my back. "Is it because you don't want to go to the hospital?"

"Yes. Because I don't want to go to the hospital . . . and because I'll miss you both."

"Oh, we'll come and see you, Mom." Adam's voice was tender and full of self-satisfaction. He'd solved the problem. They'd come and see me.

"Great idea," I said kissing his eyes, his cheeks, his chin. "And I'll call you a lot, honey. Okay? Okay, Todd? If Mommy calls you up will you talk to me on the telephone?" Todd grinned his "the-devil-made-me-do-it" grin, and said "Yes, Mommy-Moomy-Mommy."

"Mommy moomy mommy. You can't take that away from me," I sang, with my best Frank Sinatra phrasing.

As I threw nightgowns and toilet articles into a small suitcase, I thought about how I'd packed for the hospital when Adam was born. Weeks too early, of course, and with a myopic attention to detail.

Having dutifully uttered all of the prenatal clichés—"We don't care if it's a boy or a girl, as long as it's healthy"—we secretly believed that if you said that, what you were bound to receive was, at best, a healthy leftover. If you said you were having a boy, Neill would say patting my belly, you would have a boy. But only if you really believed it. He really believed it.

I, on the other hand, was determined to remain noncommittal down to the last detail. So when I packed my three brand-new nightgowns, I carefully laid the blue on the left side of the suitcase, the pink on the right side, and over both the neutral white. When Neill learned he had a son, he attributed it to the power of positive thinking. I, of course, knew better—the white nightgown had blue ribbon around the cuffs.

Packing for brain surgery required a different but no less superstitious strategy. I threw in every piece of jewelry that meant anything to me: rings Neill had given me at each of the boys' births; the mezuzah Jack's wife had taken from around her own neck the night before. Then my favorite books: Saul Bellow's *Herzog* and William Styron's *Lie Down in Darkness*. At the last moment I added *The Collected Works of Edna St. Vincent Millay*; I didn't want or need all of the poems, just "Renascence."

As we drove silently along the parkway, our hands gripped together, the third-rate lyricist in me would not be still. Music from *Sweet Charity* floated in and out of my water-bound brain.

"If they could see us now," I hummed, stroking Neill's face. Not the part about the gorgeous clothes or drinkin' fancy wine. No, that was irrelevant. It was the song's finish I couldn't shake loose. "If my friends could see me now . . . they'd never believe it. If my friends could see me now."

Here we were, I thought, everybody's candidates for the Golden Couple Award, wending our way toward hell.

BEING ADMITTED TO THE HOSPITAL WAS CURIOUSLY COMFORTING. This was not a new feeling. Plunk me down on one of those turquoise or orange Naugahyde chairs that are omnipresent in hospitals; set me opposite a clerk who never looks up; let that clerk roll a crisp white form into the typewriter, and I am immediately enveloped by a childlike sense of well-being. I have made it. I have arrived at the place. Here I will not only be taken care of, I will be taken seriously. Everything I say, do, and even hint at will be recorded. In triplicate, at least. What harm can possibly come to me here that I am not protected against?

Take me, Neurological Institute; I am yours. Perhaps the pleasurable relief I experienced that mid-June day was owing to my prior hospital admissions.

Two obstetrical admissions—nobody who waits nine months to enter the hospital isn't glad to be there. In both cases I arrived hours too soon, feeling strong and confident. I was made up, coiffed, manicured, and even pedicured. (I was certain there would be a moment, mid-delivery, when the obstetrician would look up and notice those feet. "Oh my gosh!" he'd shriek, "will you look at those feet! Have you ever seen anything more gorgeous!" It would have been worth all of the contortions necessary to get Misty Mocha nail polish past the protruberance of a nine-month-old fetus for that one moment of pedicled glory.)

Wearing my Christmas red maternity pantsuit, I had looked more like a guest at a holiday buffet than a woman in advanced labor on the February morning in 1970 when I was admitted to Chicago's Michael Reese Hospital. The fact that one bright red pant leg was soaked with amniotic fluid didn't slow me down a bit. It was simply my ticket of admission; it proved that in spite of my good humor and pain-free expression, I belonged there.

I had had such a good time being admitted for Adam's birth that

28

when it was time to get Todd's show on the road, I had the same red suit dry-cleaned twice and wore it again. In part, it was a superstitious effort to duplicate the trouble-free birth of my first baby. But it was also true that Adam had been born in Chicago; they hadn't yet seen this dazzling display in New York. There was a whole new audience waiting at Mount Sinai three and a half years later.

Maternity admissions are unique; they offer pain rewarded. No other hospital admissions are so joyous.

Well, joyous had been done—twice. My next admission, for emergency abdominal surgery, had another character entirely.

I awoke one morning in January 1975, to a brisk New York snowfall and a mildly aching belly. Neill was in California, on one of his monthly business trips to visit the West Coast companies in his portfolio. Through a morning's chores, the discomfort didn't go away, but neither did the children's plaintive litany, "When can we go out and play in it? Mommy? When?"

"When it stops," I kept saying. They thought I meant the snowfall; I, however, meant the pain. It wasn't getting any worse, but it wasn't getting any better, either. I briefly considered a call to an internist I had seen only once, and then for a routine physical. Since it was unlikely that he would recognize my name, I dismissed the idea of calling him. To hell with it, I thought, looking out the window at four inches of snow; in New York City that's a traffic stopper for sure. Getting from Riverdale to the doctor's midtown Manhattan office and back would be much more difficult than enduring a stomachache.

"Get out the mittens and boots, kids. We're going sledding." It was only when I doubled up after the third run down the hill that another mother-sledder insisted I call the doctor.

"Neill's away," she said logically through clouds of frosted breath. "What'll you do if you have to call the doctor at three in the morning instead of three in the afternoon? Hmm? Where are you going to get a baby-sitter then?" Adam and Todd were already half soaked with the snow, and the cold was getting to them as fast as the pain was getting to me.

"Time to pack it in, guys," I said. " 'Sesame Street' will be on soon." Nobody argued.

"I can't diagnose a bellyache over the phone," said the internist, whose name it had taken me nearly half an hour to recall. "Meet me at the emergency room at Mount Sinai at five o'clock."

29

"Isn't this a killer?" I said to the balding taxi driver who was cursing the Major Deegan Expressway. The Deegan is no Indy 500 at 4 P.M. on a summer's day either, but this day offered an endless gray vista of the Bronx passing by in agonizingly slow motion. Gray sky, gray air, gray buildings, gray people behind the wheels of their nearly motionless cars.

"Yeah," the driver muttered, "a killer." An often neglected aspect of being a New Yorker who isn't a native is to take such rejoinders as his "yeah, a killer" for New York City taxi-driver wit. It's just another way in which outsiders are vulnerable in the Big Apple. Besides, I had no one else to talk to.

"I mean, I'm on my way to the hospital for GodKnowsWhat, my kids are home with a babysitter who can't cook, and it's almost dinnertime. My husband's in California. All I've got with me is a toothbrush and a Blue Cross card. What do you think?"

"Yeah, it's a killer, all right."

When the driver eased the cab into a sea of slush in front of the emergency room entrance to Mount Sinai, it was ten after five.

"Yeah, well, good luck," he said, laying my change in my hand. I sat motionless staring at the busy entrance. I could see the patients inside lined up on folding chairs, sitting beneath the blue-white haze of fluorescent lights. I found it impossible to move from the cab.

"You getting out, Lady, or what?" the driver said impatiently. A young black man on crutches was waiting for the cab.

"I'm getting out," I answered. The evening air felt wet and menacing against my face.

The emergency room was a scene worthy of Goya. Whole families leaned on one another in positions so pathetic it was impossible to determine which person was the patient. Children were sobbing, some with pain, others with boredom. People slept, and cried, and paced the narrow aisle between rows of chairs. Over all of this miseryscape lay a grimy patina of fatigue—the weariness of those who must wait and wait and wait before they will know comfort.

I am so much luckier, I thought, as I checked in at the admitting desk. In moments, my fancy Park Avenue doctor materialized and led me to an examining room, away from those who could not afford private medical care. Me with my Blue Cross card and my warm fur coat.

"It's not fair," I said while a nurse drew blood for a white count to determine whether or not this was a clear case of appendicitis. The pain in my middle tightened its grip as she withdrew the needle from my arm.

"Lots of people have their appendix out, Mrs. Bernstein."

"*Brownstein*. That's not what I mean. I mean it's not fair that I just march right into an examining room while those people sit for hours waiting to be seen."

"Oh. Yeah . . . that. Well, what are you going to do? It's the American way."

I lay back on the slippery leather examining table and thought about the American way while Doctor Fancy pressed on my stomach. Again, I couldn't recall his name.

"Here?" he kept asking while I held my breath waiting for him to isolate the pain. "Here?"

"Yiiii!" I trilled when he'd scored the bull's-eye. "There!" My breath came out with a whooshing noise.

"Okay," he said, looking at his watch. "I think we've found the problem. Now, I'm going to press on that spot again, and this time I want you to tell me which hurts more: when I press, or when I let go. Ready?"

"Ready," I whispered. What an utterly unattractive man I thought, while he pressed with both hands. He should trim the hair in his ears. Someone ought to tell him that.

"Son of a bitch!" I shouted, when he let go.

"You can get dressed," he said. "I'm going to line up a surgeon. We'll wait for the white count, of course, but I'd bet my reputation there's a red-hot appendix in there. I'll go get you admitted." He was washing his well-manicured hands in a small sink.

"Just like that?" I asked, sitting up. "Bim. Bam. Boom. Surgery? Just like that? I was out sledding three hours ago, for God's sake."

"You were a fool," he said. "Now get dressed and meet me at the desk."

"Wait a minute," I said. I'd spotted a shiny black telephone on the bare white wall. "Can I use that phone? My husband's out of town and my baby-sitter thinks I'll be home any minute."

"Here," he said, reaching into the pocket of his camel's-hair sportscoat and coming up with a handful of silver. "There's a row of pay phones out in the hall. That phone is for doctors' use only. See you at the desk," he said airily.

Screw you and the horse you rode in on, buddy, I thought as I reached for the black phone.

31

There was no question about who to dial: my friend Linda. Not only was Linda my neighbor on the fourteenth floor, she was the one friend everyone should have when making an illegal phone call from an emergency room in a New York City hospital. Linda is the quintessential "big town handler."

"I can handle it" was her motto, her trademark. No matter that inside her ninety-five-pound child-woman body the Jewish princess and the Jewish mother were locked in an endless struggle for supremacy. She could handle it.

"Linda," I had said as quickly as I could, "I'm in the emergency room. At Mount Sinai. It looks like I'm going to have an appendectomy. Maybe something more serious. Yes," I said, "tonight. Go to my house and get rid of the baby-sitter. You take care of the kids, please. Then find Neill's itinerary and locate him in California. Tell him to get on the first plane heading east. Got all that?" I was breathless; she was undaunted.

"Got it. Who's doing the surgery? See if you can get Kraft. He's the best. General surgery, that is. If it's anything more specialized, call me right back and I'll tell you—"

"Linda, I'm not even supposed to be using this phone! Don't worry about who the surgeon is. Just get the kids and make sure you find my husband."

"Good-bye. I'll handle it." Click.

The doctor in the camel's-hair coat, whose name I'd forgotten again, was coming into the room just as I replaced the receiver. He was furious.

"I can't believe it," he shouted, "I simply can't believe it! There are no beds! You're going to have to go to Doctors' Hospital. Dr. Golden will meet you there. I cannot believe it." Linda probably could have gotten me a bed, but I didn't say so.

"Who's Dr. Golden?" I asked while I struggled into my panty-hose. "And would you mind closing the door?" Two orderlies were watching the show. He ignored the request and began a staccato monologue.

"He's a very competent surgeon. A Mount Sinai guy. Don't worry. And your white count, by the way, is sky high. I just can't believe it. Can you hurry up? It's rush hour out there. A cab is going to have a hell of a time getting across town." He already had his coat and hat on.

"Are you going with me?" I asked as he hailed a cab on Madi-

32

son Avenue. The fact that taxi drivers seemed to have more influence on my case than my doctor did was beginning to irritate me.

"I'll meet you there," he said, putting me into a cab that had bathed us both with icy water as it braked.

"Listen," he said sternly to the young Puerto Rican driver, "I am a doctor. Now I want you to take this young woman to Doctors' Hospital. At once! And no matter what she tells you, don't let her eat, drink, or smoke anything along the way. Is that clear? You are to take her directly to Doctors' Hospital. York Avenue. Right across from Gracie Mansion." He slammed the taxi's door.

"Whatsa matter, honey?" the driver said, looking over his shoulder. "He act like he afraid I gonna kidnap you."

"Oh no. It isn't that. He's just worried that I'm going to ditch him. It's not such a bad idea, actually," I said, lighting a forbidden cigarette.

"What's your name, driver?" I asked as we inched across Park Avenue. The snow had stopped, the temperature had risen, and New York was left to pray for a sunny tomorrow that might dry up the slop that filled the potholes. Chicago has garbage trucks to pick up snow, Minneapolis has first-rate snow removal equipment and New York City has faith. It's cheaper.

"Edouardo," the driver said politely.

"Edouardo, have you ever taken anyone to Doctors' Hospital?"

"Oh yes," he said brightening. "I been there a lot of times, miss. I know that place real good. I even took a famous person there."

"No kidding. Who?"

"Well, I don't know if I should talk about it." We were almost to Lexington Avenue. Only four more blocks.

"Come on, Edouardo. It will take my mind off my pain."

"Okay. I tell you," he said sympathetically. "It was Cher."

"Cher? You mean Sonny and Cher? That Cher?"

"That's the one," he said and then hummed a few bars of "I Got You, Babe."

"What was she there for?" I asked. I had a vision of Cher dressed in a hospital gown trimmed with red sequins and bugle beads.

"Oh, I don't know what I should say about that, miss. That's pretty personal, you know."

"Okay, don't tell me, Edouardo." He was silent a moment.

33

"I tell you. She was getting her . . . how you say it . . . her . . . chest . . . bigger. That's pretty personal, huh?"

"It certainly is," I said. It hurt when I laughed.

When the cab pulled up in front of Doctors' Hospital, Edouardo opened the door for me and I overtipped him. I was almost inside when he called out to me.

"Hey, miss! Don't let them make yours bigger. They look just fine how they are!"

"Thank you," I said, and admitted myself for surgery.

By the time they were rolling me down the hall on a gurney, Linda had arrived, assured me that my children were being cared for, interrogated the surgeon, and determined that he was worthy of taking a scalpel to my tender flesh. But just barely.

"It's not a simple appendectomy, you know," she whispered to me. "You screamed too loud when they gave you the pelvic exam. He's going in there full tilt. No bikini scar. A full exploratory. The rip-off artist!" she hissed.

She probably had more to say, lots more, but the Demerol got to me before she did.

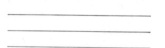

It had been only eighteen months between that hospital admission and the one today at Neuro, but that was long enough for Linda and me to have grown apart. We had had what earlier generations called a "falling out"—no genuine argument, just a mutual backing off process.

I excused myself from the office of the admitting clerk and went to a pay phone in the lobby. Neill could fill in the dates of my hospitalizations; I had a score to settle. I sat down in the phone booth, closed the folding door, and dialed my friend.

"Linda? It's Karen. Please listen to me carefully. I don't want you to talk, I just want you to listen. I'm at Neurological Institute—that's part of Columbia Presbyterian. I'm going to have brain surgery. My headaches were more serious than anyone realized . . . I may have a brain tumor." I was beginning to cry and the crying was intensifying the pain in my head. "Linda? Please don't *you* cry. Just try to listen to me. I've thought about my life long enough to realize that I owe you an apology . . . so if I've hurt you or mistreated you in any way, I want you to know . . . I'm sorry."

On the other end of the line Linda was making choking sounds.

"I don't want to talk any more now," I said. "I just wanted you to know that. Okay?"

"Okay," she sobbed. "Oh my God! Karen!"

We both hung up. I took two aspirin from the purse-size container I carried with me at all times and washed them down at the drinking fountain outside the phone booth. Then I walked back across the lobby to the admitting office.

Neill was rattling off the details of my stay at Doctors' Hospital when I walked back in.

"My goodness," said the admitting clerk, typing the information onto the form. "You certainly have had a busy medical history."

"Busy?" I echoed. "I wouldn't say busy, would you, Neill?"

"Eventful," Neill said. "Benignly eventful." He kissed my nose with cold lips. Then quickly, he switched gears.

"Would it be possible to get in touch with Dr. Mount from your office?" he asked the clerk. "If it's possible, we'd like him to operate on Karen."

Lester Mount is the extraordinary neurosurgeon who'd gained recognition as a young man through John Gunther's enduring tale of his son's fatal brain tumor, *Death Be Not Proud*. Dr. Mount had been deeply involved in Johnny Gunther's case, and was fondly and respectfully portrayed by Gunther in the book he wrote as a memorial to his son.

"Do you know Dr. Mount?" the clerk asked with reverence. The man was legendary in his profession.

"He operated on our son two years ago," Neill said matter-of-factly.

"He could be our family neurosurgeon," I said with utterly false bravado. Neill elbowed me into silence. Silence knocked me back two years to when we'd taken three-month-old Todd to Dr. Mount for a birth defect our pediatrician had spotted at Todd's first check-up.

Where the bones of an infant's skull are meant to be open in order to accommodate the growth of the brain—the place we call "the soft spot"—Todd's bones had closed. The closure was only a millimeter or two long, but that was enough to mean his head would have been misshapen. Rather like a football in profile.

"Think of it as cosmetic surgery," said our droll pediatrician, Dr. Jerry Jacobs. "You can either put a hole in his head now— and remember that Dr. Mount designed this procedure and has been doing it for twenty-five years with stunning success—or you can let him grow up with an ugly head.

"Consider it the way you would a nose job," he said.

"I would never consider a nose job for an infant," I said. My voice trembled.

"You would if his nose were ugly enough and the operation was designed to be done most effectively at three and a half months."

"Wait a minute," I asked, reeling. "Are you talking about an ugly head, a head that a good, thick head of hair like mine or Adam's will cover? Or are you talking about a grotesque head?"

"Grotesque," he said, pausing, "is in the eye of the beholder."

Dr. Jacobs had earned my trust for his candor and my respect for his diagnostic ability; so in a five-hour procedure in the winter of 1973, Dr. Lester Mount, who is known for performing operations that last fourteen to sixteen hours without ever leaving the operating room, gave Todd the perfectly round head nature had not provided.

And so the world-famous Dr. Mount, a man who looks like a Norman Rockwell rendering of a neurosurgeon, who has a profile so clean that it borders on the patrician, who makes airplanes out of rubber bands and tongue depressors for child patients, and who writes follow-up letters to the referring pediatricians that begin, "Thank you for sending me this delightful little patient," had everything to do with why I was so calm the Thursday morning I was admitted at Neuro.

"I'll call Dr. Marks and see if she can request Dr. Mount," the clerk said.

THE OVERWHELMING UGLINESS OF MY ROOM AT NEUROLOGICAL INSTITUTE gave visual consistency to my ordeal; the setting fit my plot as well as the moors of *Wuthering Heights* served Emily Brönte. The walls, which may once have been pale gray, were now the color of long-abandoned cottage cheese. The two scrawny metal beds and a small night table listing precariously between them seemed fittings more appropriate to an insane asylum. The grimy glass of the solitary window provided a fuzzy view of a room exactly like my own across a narrow court.

"Are all the rooms the same?" I asked the prim, gray-haired nurse who had accompanied me to the fifth floor while Neill was out trying to find a parking place that wasn't in a tow-away zone.

"No," she said with finality, "some aren't as nice."

My room did offer some small advantages, however: the second bed was empty and there was a telephone on the spindly night table.

"Does that phone work?" I asked doubtfully.

"Well, yes. Of course," she said. The woman was in her mid-fifties, and from the exasperated tone of her voice I gathered she'd been at Neuro long enough to have her little defense well rehearsed.

"Look, dear," she said with an acid smile, "around here we mostly save lives and find new ways to save lives. At this hospital money is spent on research, not frills." Harumph! That ought to show me.

What, exactly, had I expected? The Waldorf? Doctors' Hospital, where meals were served by white-gloved waiters? No, this was another place entirely; no nonsense, no frills. Around here we mostly save lives.

"Thank you," I said. "Do you suppose I might have something

for a headache?" I could not remember if I had taken aspirin after calling Linda or merely thought about taking them.

"Dr. Marks will be here in a little while. She'll order something for you, I'm sure. In the meantime, why don't you get settled and put this gown on." It was not a question; it was a command. My tenuous grip on my civilian status here was slipping. Once I took off my pastel summer dress and put on the hospital gown, I'd be subject to the terrifyingly serious business of having my life saved. Whatever that meant.

I began slowly to unbutton my dress.

"That's a good girl," the nurse said. "You get comfortable and I'll be right back."

I sat down on the bed, my dress unbuttoned, my feet dangling, and tried to think. The pain behind my eyes was like two steel blades twisting through my skull. I pressed my eyelids with my fingertips, as though I could push the pain back. Force it out of my head. Now that I knew it was all that fluid causing the pain, I had a very real sense of liquid sloshing around in there, pressing, pushing against my skull from within. I tried to hold my head very still to keep the tides even.

Thinking hurt. Thinking that I might no longer be able to think—that hurt worse.

Once, when Neill and I had had to cancel plans for a small dinner party because of one of my headaches, I'd teased him: "Honey, if this turns out to be not just a sinus headache or tension head-ache, but something horrible like a brain tumor, promise me you'll water me every day."

He'd promised, secure against the possibility that anything so preposterous could happen.

It was happening! He might have to water me every day. I might not be able to think. Ask questions. Read books. Care for my chil-dren. Speak. Write. If there was a brain tumor hiding behind that cloud of fluid on my CAT scan pictures, all of that could happen. And more—I could die.

I hadn't made any plans. Nobody would know what to do. It had never occurred to me to write anything remotely like a will. Oh, God, I had things to do! People I wanted to talk to. People I wanted to wrap my arms around. What was I doing here, letting my feet dangle?

I picked up the phone, jabbed fiercely at the button and got the operator to get me long distance—Chicago.

Calling Barbara and Irwin Jann was like calling my family. It was pure selfishness, but I wanted them with me. No matter what discomfort or inconvenience it would cause them to leave three young children and pause in the ongoing struggle of their marital woes, I wanted them.

Neill came into the room just as Barbara answered on the second ring. He sat down on the bed beside me.

"Who are you calling?" he whispered.

"Barbara and Irwin. Oh, Neill, I want them here. Here—you talk." I handed him the receiver and got under the covers. I was a patient now.

Barbara and Irwin had been our special friends since college. Both of them were only children who invested themselves in their friendships without restraint. Through many years of shared experience—college, graduate school, weddings, births, and vacations—Barbara had become the sister I'd always wished for and Irwin became the brother that Neill lacked.

On my twenty-seventh birthday the Brownsteins and the Janns had been in Paris together, living it up. Irwin, a thriving Chicago attorney and the cleverest man I've ever known, ordered bottle after bottle of the finest champagne and we got wildly drunk, toasting each other's successes and the promise of the future.

Late that night, dancing down the rue de la Paix, we agreed that when we got home—they to Chicago, and we to New York— we would do something to legitimize the glorious feeling we shared for each other: we'd all write wills that made us the legal guardians of each other's children. It was the adult equivalent of becoming blood brothers.

"They'll be here late this afternoon," Neill said, hanging up. He hugged me and kissed me gently. "That's from Barbara."

"Well!" boomed Melinda Marks, pretending to knock on the door, "the famous world traveler. Mr. Brownstein, I presume?"

"Neill," I said, rolling over without breaking our embrace, "this is Dr. Marks. If everyone around here does the kind of work this place is famous for, you'll be reading about Dr. Marks in my book some day."

"What's that supposed to mean?" she asked, tossing her hair. I wiggled out of Neill's arms and sat up on the edge of the bed.

"Have you forgotten, Dr. Marks? I'm a writer. And, well, I think *Death Be Not Proud* has been the ultimate brain tumor book for too long. Don't you?"

"I thought you write comedy," Dr. Marks replied without missing a beat. My headache was nearly gone and I began to sense a return to the easy banter of our first meeting.

"I do, I do write comedy, Doctor. But I'm quite versatile, and in this case, well, I think I'd settle for a good ol' happy ending. How about it, Dr. Marks, do you think you and your troops here can come up with a happy ending?" She ignored that question.

"How come you're not in a hospital gown yet?" she said breezily.

Breezy was Dr. Marks's style—studied breezy, but breezy nonetheless.

"We're holding out for the bridal suite," Neill said. He could do breezy himself, when pressed.

Melinda Marks introduced the members of her group, including Betsy, who had the courage to ask how I was feeling, and then she suggested that Neill step outside with her while I made myself look more like a patient than a visitor.

The moment Neill and Dr. Marks left me alone in that grimy, barren room, the Suspicion Demons were born in me. I, a woman who believed that trust was the cornerstone of my marriage, became instantly convinced that Neill was deceiving me. It's a conspiracy, I thought, as cold sweat began to trickle down my sides.

The focus of my mistrust was distinct and sharp: they weren't telling me everything. It was obvious—why else would they have left the room? The scenario of what was transpiring outside my door came to me with perfect clarity.

I was going to die and Neill and Melinda Marks were out there concocting a plan to keep that diagnosis from me as long as possible. The surgery was to be a hoax, a maneuver to take me off the scent of my impending doom. The shunt was only a pretense. Why else had everyone so carefully avoided mentioning the tumor this morning? It must be too late.

How often had terminal patients undergone surgery that was no more than an elaborate ruse to keep them from the unbearable truth? The procedure was so common it even had its own euphemism: "They opened him and closed him." Meaning—too late. Too bad. Hopeless. And where did that leave the patient? Dying in a pool of ignorance. How dare anyone—Neill, or Dr. Marks, or anyone—keep me from knowing my own fate?

Whatever their motives, and even in my advancing fury I made a small attempt to consider those motives, their duplicity was unconscionable. What did it matter that Neill was lying to me out of love? Or that Mike Margolin was holding out because he was too personally involved? And as for breezy Bo Peep, she was the guilt-

40

iest of them all! Where was all of yesterday's brutal candor this morning? Hmm? "Yes, it's possible you may die soon," she had said. What was that? Just a slip-up? A matter of being caught off guard? Today she was treating me like a tonsillectomy.

A decision had been reached behind my back: "Keep Karen from knowing."

"I think you have that gown on backwards, honey," Neill said when he came back in. He was smiling at me. His smile only confirmed my theory. What could be more suspicious than his smiling at this moment? I was going to have brain surgery, what the hell was he smiling for?

"What did she say?" I asked, fighting hysteria. "Tell me exactly what she said, Neill. Exactly. Word for word." He took off his jacket and loosened his tie.

"She said you'd have some tests today, and maybe tomorrow, and that the surgery would probably be sometime tomorrow afternoon."

He sat down on the empty bed and stared into the court, past me.

"That's not all she said, dammit. You were out there a good ten minutes! Look at me! I want to know everything!" The blades were twisting behind my eyes again. I covered my eyes with a pillow.

"We talked about Dr. Mount . . ."

"And?"

"And, unfortunately, Dr. Mount is addressing some prestigious gathering of neurosurgeons tomorrow." He sighed.

"That's swell," I said, dropping the cool, white pillow and letting my frustration run full steam at Neill.

"That's just perfect. No bridal suite. No Dr. Mount. No nothing. Perfect!"

"Dr. McMurtry is going to do the operation," Neill said as calmly as a man under attack from all sides could possibly have spoken. "He's a wonderful neurosurgeon. Younger than Dr. Mount, but just as skilled. They office together."

"Yes. Right. I remember," I said bitterly. "How chummy. And besides, it's just bread-and-butter surgery, anyway. Funny how you can keep forgetting that when it's your brain they're going to spread on their toast." I was crying now, making no attempt to control my paranoia.

"Karen," Neill said sharply, "if you don't stop this right now, I am going to walk out of this room!" His anger silenced me, calmed me somehow. Like a slap across the face.

41

"Jim McMurtry is a first-rate man. You're lucky to have him. Now cut out all this bitchiness. It isn't making things any easier. Not for me or for you."

He was right, of course. This was no time for histrionics.

Dr. Marks and her troops returned to examine me and take my history. She repeated almost verbatim the questions she had asked only twenty-four hours before, but with none of the Wedgwood-blue flair of the first interrogation. This interview was strictly instructional: Suspected Brain Tumors 101. Take notes.

"Ever have nausea?"

"No. Never."

"Vomiting?"

"No."

"Blurred vision?"

"Once."

"Ever faint?"

"No."

"Lose your balance?"

"No."

"Have seizures?"

"Oh, no!"

"Loss of memory?"

"Not that I can remember."

"Ever black out?"

"No."

"Ever have trouble thinking of the right word?"

"Is that a serious question or a slur on my credentials as a writer?"

"A serious question. Do you ever know what you want to say, but the words won't come?" Her eyes never left the clipboard.

"You got me, Dr. Marks," I confessed.

I'd stopped writing about six months before, blocked in a way I had never experienced before. For the first time in my life I was filling pages with words that meant nothing, not even to me. I tore things up as fast as I wrote them. It was all garbage, nothing worth salvaging at all.

"Ever see double?"

"You asked me that yesterday," I said, beginning to resent my role as a case study. "You know the answer."

"Yes, but they don't," she said coldly, indicating her flock. I was an obstacle to learning. The nerve of me.

"I had double vision last night. For the first time."

"How about that," she said with a grin. And she took a few notes of her own.

"Now, would you tell us about the headaches, Karen?"

The troops came to attention. Even the bleary-eyed residents who'd been sneaking covetous looks at the empty bed.

I repeated everything I could remember saying the day before. How I'd had a history of sinus headaches. How the intranasal injections has ceased to be effective in thwarting pain. How the headaches were brief, but intense. How over time their frequency had increased. How the pain was there when I woke up in the morning. How for the last few weeks I couldn't lift my head from the pillow before swallowing aspirin. I gave them the straight goods—none of my usual storyteller's embellishment.

"Did the aspirin help?" someone in the back asked.

"I don't know," I answered truthfully. "Sometimes I thought it did."

"Well, did you feel relief?"

"I don't know how to answer that," I said softly. "I have a headache right now. This minute. I'd like to think that a pill could take it away. I guess that's naive, isn't it?"

God, but I was tired of talking about myself. I could bang my own drum, toot my own horn, and be a perfectly worthy center of attention for almost anything, if only it didn't have to be this.

"You're so special," people had been telling me all my life. Parents, teachers, boyfriends, scholarship committees, employers. And maybe the worst part was that in retrospect, I agreed. I had it all. The happy childhood, the carefree adolescence, the popularity so sought after in youth, the happy marriage, the creative satisfaction of my work, the healthy kids.

But special was supposed to mean exceptional, not peculiar. Special was supposed to mean "gee, I wish I was like her," not "how extraordinary, poor thing!"

So MANY WHITE-COATED INTERROGATORS HAD VISITED MY ROOM by noon on the next day that I suggested to Neill that we post a hand-lettered sign on the door:

GO AWAY

STOP ASKING ME QUESTIONS

COME BACK WHEN YOU HAVE ANSWERS

In a teaching hospital, medical students, interns, and especially first-year residents are drawn to an interesting case like flies to a picnic. Their learning fattens on people like me.

"Have you checked out the new stuff in Room 403?" I could imagine them whispering to each other in the corridors. "You really ought to stop by *that* one," they'd say.

And stop by they did. Neill and I would just be easing into a careful conversation about how we should readjust our moving plans when a new swarm would come buzzing through the door.

They were polite flies, I have to admit. They never picked at me without asking permission first. The students and interns, bright-eyed and embarrassingly eager, never forgot to thank me for the opportunity I'd provided them. The fact that their appreciation was usually expressed immediately after they'd peered into my eyes drove me wild. Melinda Marks's comment about never having seen so much papilledema in a patient who wasn't comatose haunted me.

"I guess you guys hit pay dirt with me," I said when the last in a group of four put down his opthalmoscope and stepped back.

44

"Excuse me, ma'am?" said the curly-haired, nervous young man. He looked around in confusion for a sign from his peers.

"My eyes," I said with perverse pleasure. "All that papilledema. Have you ever seen anything like that before?" He stared at me blankly.

"Uh, no ma'am," he said, backing away. And they were gone, all of them, in a hushed chorus of thank yous, leaving Neill and me to agonize over why I should be so popular a patient on the fourth floor.

"Put on a robe," Neill finally said. "Let's go on a little reconnaissance mission."

"Get the lay of the land?"

"Right," he said, helping me on with a flowered ankle-length number that was more hostess gown than hospital robe.

"And besides," he added, kissing the back of my neck, "if they find your bed empty, all those good-looking young doctors will have to find somebody else to grill for a while."

"Good-looking, my ass," I said, as we stepped tentatively out into the hall. "They all give me the creeps."

We held hands and strolled down the dark green linoleum hall. Innocents abroad. Heading for the Tivoli Gardens, we had mistakenly bungled our way into the House of Usher.

A totally bald woman pushed her wheelchair directly into our path; the outline of a steel plate under her scalp was clearly visible as she rolled past. Behind her came a young man, his youth stolen by the white bandages that swathed his head. With a trembling hand he reached out to touch the guard rails along the wall.

He grinned shyly at me, that young man, and nodded. I wanted so to look away, pretend I didn't see him. Instead, summoning courage against all odds, I self-consciously smiled back at him across an ocean of terror. He knew what lay in the distance between us; I could only wonder.

"Nice day," he said weakly when we came abreast. He could not have been more than eighteen or nineteen. "Not too hot." I squeezed my wet palm against Neill's hand.

"Right," I said. "Not too hot at all." We walked on. Somehow it was necessary to make it to the end of the hall, not give in to the dread that was creeping through every part of my body. Keep going. Past room after room of shaved heads, mummied skulls, we went on. When we reached the end of the hall, there was a small empty bench.

"Sit down," Neill said. His face, distorted as if by the pain I was suffering, was a mask of fear. Had he too visualized my face under those white helmets?

"No. My head hurts. I want to go back," I whispered. "I can't handle this. Neill, please let's go back!" I didn't wait for an answer. I fled.

Away from the bandaged heads, the hand rails, the wheelchairs, the walking wounded. Away from the awareness that I, simply by sharing this grotesque space with them, was one of them. Away from Neill and the awful truth of this day.

In front of my room there was a gurney, a body cart. Lying on the cart was a pretty, black-haired woman in her mid-thirties with the eyes of a gypsy dancer. She propped her head on one elbow and looked me over.

"Are you Karen?" she asked, hopefully.

"Yes. How did you know my name?"

"I've been looking for you all over the fourth floor," she said cheerfully. "Dr. Marks thinks we might have something in common. I know you're a "brain" and I'm a "back," but I'm hoping we can overcome those barriers." She laughed, a full-throated sexy laugh. "Dr. Marks told me you're a writer; I'm an artist."

She reached down to a side pocket on the cart and showed me her small sketchbook. Only then did I notice that she couldn't move her lower body.

"My name is Ruth," she said, reaching out with a well-muscled arm to shake my hand. "Maybe we can be friends."

"Did anyone ever tell you that you look like Elizabeth Taylor, Ruth?" I asked, amazed at my ability to make small talk with a half-paralyzed stranger.

"Around here they say so. But then again, around here they're pretty desperate. I guess you've noticed."

"Well, it's not exactly where the Beautiful People hang out, but—"

"But nothing," she said firmly. "It's the pits. Take it from me; I'm a native. I've been here three times in the last year, and this time it's going on two months."

"Do you have a famiily?" I asked. We were chatting. My God, we were chatting.

"Three kids," she said, "and a husband who's better than all of Elizabeth Taylor's husbands put together—and a mother and father who look after the kids while I lie here waiting for a miracle."

What a wonderful speech, I thought—not just the words she

had spoken, but the way in which she had spoken them. There was no bitterness. No anger. No "Why me?" self pity. "I wait for a miracle," she'd said. It was the straightest line I'd ever heard.

"We *are* going to be friends, Ruth," I told her. "There's plenty of room in my life here for a new friend." It was like childhood, so simple, so full of trust:

"Hey, you wanna be friends?"

"Yeah, let's be friends."

She gave me her room number, took back her sketchbook, and asked me to visit her later in the day.

"Be sure to wear your blinders," she said as I pushed her down the hall. "Carry them with you whenever you leave your room. This is a pre- and post-operative floor. That means there are no scenic routes between your room and mine. I suppose you've noticed."

"I've noticed." We had come to the nurses' station in the center of the hallway.

"Mrs. Brownstein?" the prim nurse who'd admitted me called out. "You can have your aspirin now. And Dr. McMurtry is on the floor. He'll want to see you. Better get back to your room, young lady."

"Yes, ma'am. On the double." I swallowed the tablets and gave her a crisp salute.

"See you later, Brain," Ruth called out.

"Sure thing, Back," I replied.

———————————
———————————
———————————

Brains and backs, I thought as I walked briskly down the hall, looking nowhere, seeing nothing. "The house of hopes and horrors." What do they do around here for comic relief? Suddenly I remembered a phone call we'd had from Dr. Mount when Todd was in intensive care in this building, two years ago.

"This is Dr. Mount calling," a friendly voice had announced on the third morning after Todd's operation. "You had better come over here right away and pick up your baby. The nurses are spoiling him rotten."

And no wonder. Except for the tiny gauze bandage at the top of his head, he was as bright as the morning star. Pink and smiling, Todd was the most wonderfully healthy child those nurses had cared for in weeks. They fought over who would change his diaper

47

and begged to give him one last feeding before we took him home. Neill and I had been punch-drunk when we left the building with Todd—high on normalcy.

There was a curious etiquette functioning in this macabre atmosphere; what I was picking up on as I walked these halls, nodding and smiling to other patients now, were the unspoken rules of the house: keep your nightmare to yourself. You don't mess with my terrors, I'll stay away from yours. Smile. Nod. Mention the weather. But don't ask questions. Don't risk hearing the answers.

It was no accident that Ruth had not asked me what exactly was wrong with my brain, and it had been enough for me to see her lush body immobile to keep me from probing her case.

Whatever comic relief I might look forward to in this place I'd either have to import from outside the stone walls or manufacture myself with whatever resources were still left to me. Could I manage that, I wondered, as I approached my room. Could I still be funny? When all of this was over, would I be able to write comedy again? Make people laugh? Make myself laugh? All of the tampering that might be done with my brain would be acceptable to me, I thought, so long as that one precious escape valve—humor—was left intact.

The chief tamperer was waiting for me in my room.

"Mrs. Brownstein," he said in a sure, mellow voice with just the merest tinge of Texas around the edges, "I'm Dr. McMurtry." I sat down on the bed opposite Neill and this broad-shouldered stranger, and tried to focus on the man who might have the answers for me.

Dr. JAMES G. MCMURTRY III IS NOT ONLY AN OUTSTANDING NEUROSURGEON; he looks like the man you'd want to send in to do one-on-one combat with the angel of Death: big, solid, and unrelentingly human. His large, meaty hands gave lie to the stereotype of his profession. This was no bespectacled gentleman with long, delicate fingers; this was a clear-eyed Paul Bunyan, minus the ox. It might just be possible, I thought, given the sparks in his blue eyes, that he would not mess with my humor hemisphere at all. He might, in fact, be able to handle the whole shooting match in a totally satisfactory way.

"I'm glad you're here," I said. "I hope I haven't kept you waiting."

"Where were you?" Neill asked, sounding like a parent whose wayward teen-ager had come home late again.

"I was out making a new friend," I said with more vigor than I felt. "I'm a people freak, Dr. McMurtry. I get high on folks."

"Well," he said, with a fine and free smile breaking across his face. "There's nothing wrong with that."

This was all the encouragement I needed from him to launch into a little self-directed personality sketch of the *real* Karen Osney Brownstein. Before he could move out the artillery of hospital jargon and level a whole woman to notes on a pad, I headed him off at the pass. If he was going to make the definitive tour of my brain, I wanted him to have a road map that offered more than the anatomical roadside attractions; I wanted my sensibilities laid out before him like a six-page color spread in *Gray's Anatomy*.

As though I were describing the treasures of Tut to the dig team about to unearth the tomb, I told Dr. McMurtry exactly what he could expect to find in the darker regions. It took more time than

I would have guessed to say what might have been reduced to a simple "please save my life with no expense to my mind."

I felt a compulsion to convince him that my brain was worth saving. How could I do that? Would my official résumé have made him any more impressed with my case? Letters of recommendation from notable professors perhaps? Testimonials from audiences who'd been wildly entertained by my writing? Could these force his hand to brilliance in my behalf?

What did I really want to say to him? "This is no average bear you're dealing with; give it your best shot."

When at last all that intelligence I'd been trying so hard to demonstrate in my monologue finally came to the fore and prevented me from making a worse fool of myself than I already had, all I could say to the man was, "I'm sorry. I guess I'm just a little nervous."

"Well, sure you are," he said gently. "Of course you are." And then with a simple but powerful display of his own intelligence he added, *"Both* of you must be very worried."

I could see the appreciation bubbling up in my husband's wounded dark eyes before he spoke. But I could not have predicted what he would say.

"Dr. McMurtry," he began cautiously, "I hesitated to bring this up, but you've put me at ease enough to mention it. You may be a tall Texas stranger to Karen, but I've heard a good deal about you from your brother, Burt. He and I share some business matters."

"Please, Neill, get to the point," I said. What did this have to do with surgery?

"The point is, Burt brags about you quite a bit, Doctor. And now I know why."

"Well," said Dr. McMurtry in his slow, easy demi-drawl, "Burt's quite a guy himself."

"Yes, he is," Neill said with so much enthusiasm I feared I was about to be forgotten in the midst of all this Old Boy good will. I was wrong, though; Neill put us back on course straightaway.

"And in regard to your supposition, doctor, that we're both worried? Well, I'm afraid you've understated it. I don't mind telling you we're both scared shitless!"

Dr. McMurtry folded his arms across his chest, a gesture that enhanced his aura of solidarity.

"Well, let me see if I can't be of some help here. Let's see if I can explain a few things."

And then, in that soft-spoken, almost laconic manner that was a comfort all by itself, he began to speak of the unspeakable.

A gentleman to the core, Dr. McMurtry began by praising the work of others. Melinda Marks was a "fine" doctor, he said. "Just fine." But while he softly spoke of her competence, I could not help but think of her brusqueness. The contrast between their styles was so striking—where he was making every effort to reassure me, she had missed no opportunity to frighten me. The comparison left a huge dent in my feminism.

Quickly, Dr. McMurtry turned his attention to the CAT scan I'd had on the previous day. He explained that this computerized scan, introduced into the United States in 1973 and put into widespread use a mere two years before I had needed it, was able to provide more detailed pictures of the contents of the skull than any previous device.

"It's a truly remarkable tool," he said, his soft voice full of boyish wonder. "It allows us to look at the brain and see the ventricles."

"Ventricles?" I asked. "I thought ventricles were in the heart." My last brush with human anatomy had been as a high school student in sophomore biology. But it was an honors class, for crying out loud. Why didn't I know about ventricles in the head?

"Well, there are ventricles in your brain, too, and in your pictures, what we saw were enlarged ventricles. And that was very helpful to us. Seeing such enlarged ventricles explains your headaches and the papilledema."

Neill, who often functioned as an investor in and board member of sophisticated technological companies, seemed to be following this with perfect understanding. He knew the CAT scan on other, less personal terms than I did. To me, the machine's function was utterly mysterious.

"Forgive me for interrupting," I said uneasily, "but all this talk about enlarged ventricles does not explain my headaches to *me*."

"Of course not," said Dr. McMurtry kindly, "let me explain further."

What he provided was the short course in the anatomy of the head, a normal head. Your head, for instance.

Spinal fluid is manufactured in the lateral ventricles; it drains down the third ventricle, through the aqueduct into the fourth ventricle, and then out.

In my head, the savvy CAT scan had said, there was enlargement of the lateral and third ventricles. What enlarged ventricles meant for me was that there was a blockage in the normal pathway through which the spinal fluid drains, so my fluid was not draining, it was building up.

"That blockage," I asked deliberately, "is that blockage a tumor?" I took deep breaths while Dr. McMurtry continued in that same steady but relaxed manner he'd used to discuss his brother.

"That's possible, of course. But there are at least half a dozen other things that could be causing that fluid not to drain properly."

"Like what?" I begged, "tell me."

"Well, aqueductal stenosis for one. And there are a host of others. Let's not jump the gun on this, Mrs. Brownstein. Let's not even think about a tumor right now. There are two tests that will help us to get a better idea of why that pressure is building up."

"What is aqueductal stenosis?" Neill asked for me. I blew him a kiss over Dr. McMurtry's head.

"It's a congenital defect," he said in a way that, for him, was hurried. He clearly did not want to dwell on any specific diagnosis until more tests were done. He shuffled his feet and tried to continue, but I interrupted him again.

"Does aqueductal stenosis require surgery?" I asked. "Can it be cured?" Was it possible there was something even more deadly than a tumor that could invade the brain?

"The shunting procedure which you will have tomorrow is the usual treatment for aqueductal stenosis," he said.

"Then that's what I have, right?" If a shunt was bread-and-butter surgery and that's what I was going to have, maybe this wasn't the end of the line. Maybe my panic had been premature.

"Slow down here," he answered. "You are having the shunt installed in order to divert the cerebrospinal fluid inside your head. That procedure should reduce the size of the ventricles regardless of what is causing the blockage. A shunt is just a one-way valve and the one way is out of your brain."

I was back on square one. I was going to be shunted, no matter why. A current Linda Ronstadt song floated across my consciousness. I created the lyrics of a brand-new, heart-twanging, country/western ballad and sang it for my audience of two.

> "Ah've been shunted,
> Been affronted,
> When will ah be cured?"

52

"Clever lady, isn't she?" Dr. McMurtry said to Neill.

"That she is," said Neill proudly.

And while we were on the subject, there was one more question I wanted to ask: *clever*. Would I be clever when all this was over? When they put away their knives and their drills and their sophisticated machinery, would I still be clever?

I kept that question to myself. I'd done enough in the service of my own ego for this round.

The big event for that afternoon was to be a test called an arteriogram, a diagnostic procedure designed to shed some small light on the question of enlarged ventricles. In this case, the search was on for an abnormality in the blood vessels of my head. Some large lump in my arterial system might be the culprit.

Even under mild sedation, I thought, the basement of Neuro, where the test was administered, was beginning to look familiar. Just down the hall from here I'd had the CAT scan.

Where is John Ubeleski when I need him, I wondered as they wheeled me into the testing room, groggy but conscious of three or four men transferring me to a flat metal table.

Lying on my back, ordered to lie perfectly still, I had the sense of being held hostage on the set of a long-forgotten science-fiction thriller. Hulking machines were everywhere. It was difficult to tell where one of the angular machines began and another left off. In my line of sight they were an unending series of menacing forms, each with an X-ray eye: an eye focused on me with steely recognition. I could see no ceiling when I looked up, only the intricate tangle of looming machinery. My blood ran cold. Surely they'd see *that* on their precious pictures, I thought.

"This is going to be slightly uncomfortable," I heard one of those faceless men say. Not a single human detail was able to reach me while those mechanical monsters hung above.

"Are you going to use that one on me?" I asked, pointing to the large black boxlike contrivance nearest me.

"No, no. Not today," the technician said with ironic apology. "Today we're just going to insert a thin plastic catheter through the femoral artery to the aorta and take some pictures of the blood vessels in your brain. That doesn't sound too bad, does it?"

"Where's my femoral artery?" I asked.

"In your groin."

"It sounds terrible," I said. He laughed and stuck a needle in my crotch.

"You okay?" he asked in a voice as mechanical as the space that had spawned him.

"Who, me?" I said. "Super. Just super. You go right ahead and thread that thing. Just let me know when you get to my heart." Two cold tears slid down the sides of my head.

It wasn't that it was painful; it was just so terribly invasive. A thin little tube running mindlessly to my heart, dye coursing through my veins, a roomful of strangers watching me through a glass window. And a machine on the other side of the window where those strangers were on the lookout for an abnormality— *my* abnormality. Monitored by their machines, I bit my lip until I could taste blood.

When the test ended more than an hour later, my back felt as though it had spent the afternoon on a rack in some steel-walled dungeon. And what, after all, had all of those anonymous voyeurs learned from their wondrous machines?

Nothing. Zip. All they had seen was some distortion of the normal blood vessel anatomy caused by enlarged ventricles in my head. This test cost $301.00, I learned when I asked. It had failed to be instructive. A CAT scan costs $289.00. It's a better deal. All the way around.

THE ARTERIOGRAM HAD BEEN A DIAGNOSTIC BUST; I KNEW IT by the time two chattering male nurse's aides had wheeled me back to my room. Talk about your instant pictures—nowhere are the times of your life so quickly recorded as in state-of-the-art X-ray technology.

Dusk crept into the cell-like room, wrapping the miserable old walls in the only glow that might disguise them. Through the rapidly fading haze of my mild sedation, the narrow, white-sheeted hospital bed felt luxurious after my ordeal on the metal table. The thin, bleached out blanket had become the softest of down comforters. I knew I would sleep.

I awoke briefly to hear Melinda Marks saying confidently, "The pneumoencephalogram will tell it all."

"Don't buy it," I mumbled sleepily, reaching out for Neill's hand. "She said the same thing about the CAT scan." And then I dozed off again, this time into the first real sleep my body had known in thirty-six hours.

A gorgeously familiar voice woke me.

"We're here," Barbara said. She kissed me awake. My enchanted sister—I knew her perfume as well as my own. Irwin stood beside her, and for a moment I forgot where we were. I forgot that they had left the private hell their marriage had become in recent weeks to take a breather in somebody else's bad dream; forgot that this wasn't an airport arrival gate at O'Hare or JFK. For the first time in a decade, our being together was not a cause for celebration.

"Where shall we go for dinner," I said, hugging them both.

"Listen, Mama," Irwin said, blinking tears back behind his fashionable tinted glasses, "we ain't goin' nowhere until I give you the hiccups." It was our oldest and most intimate joke: no encounter between Irwin and me was complete without his wit reducing me to spasms of choked laughter.

"You did it, Irwin," I said. "Just by hinting at the possibility that you *could* do it, you've made me laugh. I'd have lost big money betting against you today."

"Well," he said, studying Barbara's expression, "it's comforting to know some things stay the same."

I ignored whatever suffering lay behind his words and her luminous hazel eyes and thanked God for their friendship while Neill hugged and kissed them both.

"Shall we cry together, or in pairs?" Irwin asked. It had been one of the consistent delights of our travels together that any way the four of us chose to split up for our day's adventures, the combinations were not only workable, but agreeable.

"In pairs," Neill suggested. Their arrival offered Neill the first genuine relief valve for his own demons; until Barbara and Irwin walked in, he had been doing his damndest to carry off the role of Man Mountain Jones.

"Let's take a walk, Ir," he said, leaving Barbara and me in the twilight.

"You look different," I said when we were alone.

"Well, you don't look so hot yourself, pal," she laughed.

"I didn't mean it that way, Barb." It was nothing I could define: her burnished auburn hair still stubbornly refused to curl around her shoulders. She was dressed, as always, with understated elegance, and bare of any jewelry except for the diamonds on her wedding ring finger. Even the small, slightly upturned nose she'd acquired through cosmetic surgery—and against Irwin's furious opposition—the year before, even that looked familiar. It wasn't her face, I decided, it was the way she held it—higher, prouder than I had ever seen before.

"I know it's getting to be a cliché, but I have to say it Barb— you look like you are your own woman."

"I'm trying, Kare, God knows I'm trying." It was an angry whisper.

Through all the years of a friendship that had begun when we were both fourteen and continued without interruption to this moment, I had never seen her so determined. Or so sad—that was it. I had never seen her sad before, so openly sad.

Barbara had always been able to cope. When Irwin began to make his move in the legal profession, Barbara quietly gave up her teaching career. And if he called her at 4 P.M. and casually an-

56

nounced he was bringing four judges home for dinner, you could bet money that when their honors walked in the door at 6 P.M. the baby would have been bathed, a gourmet meal would be simmering in the kitchen, and the Rosenthal crystal would be sparkling on the table. All of Barbara's intelligence and drive, the charm and self-confidence that had marked her career as a classroom teacher, spun one hundred and eighty degrees and turned inward, toward the family, the home. And what a home!

Every move for Barbara and Irwin had been up. Their magnificent twenty-seven-room home in Chicago's North Shore was her masterpiece, the ultimate testimonial to Barbara the coper. The consummate coper. Behind all that lovely red brick and leaded glass, she coped with three children, ten bathrooms, and one runaway ego—his. She did it all splendidly, with ease. A child of wealth, she slid gracefully into her own castle.

But now the castle walls were crumbling; she no longer loved the prince.

It all would have been so simple, the fairy tale so neatly salvaged, if the prince had only had Barbara's gift for coping, her flexibility. Instead, Irwin saw a failing marriage as the gauntlet thrown down, and if there was one thing he loved more than Baraara, it was challenge. And winning.

Winning in court rooms, winning at conference tables, winning behind the wheel of race cars; by the age of thirty-four, he had developed so keen an appetite for victory that losing a wife was unthinkable. Oh, how I wished I could help them, and how ill-equipped I was to try.

I began to feel drowsy again. "Some friend I turned out to be," I said sleepily to Barbara. "You fly eight hundred miles just to hold my hand, and I can't even stay awake long enough to ask you how things are."

"Things are rotten," she said. "And there's nothing you can do to change that, so go ahead and sleep while you can." She kicked off her shoes and stretched out on the empty bed across from mine.

Just like our high school sleepovers, I thought as I stared at the shadows on the ceiling. Just like the good old days.

"Oh, Barb," I said, pitying us both, "how did we manage to get ourselves into this mess? How did we ever get into such trouble so fast? Yesterday our most important problem was keeping our pantyhose clean and today, today—oh, dammit, Barbara, I don't want to die!"

I could hear her crying softly, but I couldn't look at her.

"Kare, I don't want you to die, either," she whispered. "If you die on me now, I'll never forgive you."

"Yes, you will, Barbara, stop talking like that." It was all so bizarre—the room, the conversation, the very fact of our being together under these circumstances; all of it had the shuddering quality of a bad dream. If only I could sleep through the next two weeks, and wake up in California with no memory of this billowing horror. If only.

"I want to talk about my children, Barbara," I said abruptly. "If you don't think you can handle it at this moment, tell me. Now. Before I get started." There were things that had to be said—things I wanted to tell my parents, and most of all things I wanted to say to Neill—but they had stuck in my throat every time I tried to begin.

I had no will, no official document or sequestered letter lying in a drawer somewhere that laid out my thoughts or wishes for Adam's and Todd's futures. All of the times Neill and I had even begun to discuss the possibility of premature death our fears had centered around Neill's frequent traveling and the prospect of a plane crash.

Mostly, such conversations had ended with tender lovemaking, and promises that we really would visit a lawyer someday soon. But those talks had been deliciously dramatic teases, the romantic playacting of lovers. The talk we needed to have now would be the real thing.

"Barbara? Are you there?"

"I'm here. Talk."

I sat up and propped the meager pillow behind me. I wanted her to see me clearly and I wanted her to remember this conversation with perfect detail—I could only say it once.

"If I die, Barbara, I expect that Neill will remarry. I don't mean to say that he won't mourn or grieve. What I do mean is that both he and I have loved our marriage enough, tasted its pleasures so thoroughly, that he may be one of the dying breed of men who understand marriage well enough to want it. And that's okay by me—provided she isn't stupid, or outrageously beautiful. I'd rather think of him being happy than sad. Whoever she is, if Neill loves her, take it on faith, and be good to her. You don't have to love her. Just let Neill know that it's all right that *he* loves her."

"Jesus, you're grown up," Barbara said. "Are you for real?"

"I think so. Just let me keep talking and then decide." I told her that I expected part of Neill's wish to remarry would come from his concern for our sons. Not the every-kid-needs-a-mother kind of concern, but rather his intense sense of family.

As I spoke, I could feel myself approaching, the long way around, the steel curtain. When I finally came to it, it was gone.

"I'm going to cry when I talk about the kids. But please, Barb, bear with me. Make sure I say it all." I leaned back and closed my eyes. Maybe it was true that Neill might not believe every child needs a mother, but *I* believe it. And I knew that he wasn't going to replace me overnight; there would be a gap, however long, when Adam and Todd were without. I wanted Barbara to fill that gap.

Considering Neill's talents as a parent, it wouldn't be all that awesome a role to fill. In all of the important matters of child rearing, I trusted Neill as well as I trusted myself. Sometimes more than I trusted myself, I told Barbara. I felt sure Neill could manage their emotional needs and intellectual concerns as a single parent. It was in the odds and ends, the trivia of raising children, that I feared he might fail them. And in some sense, me.

"Books, for example," I said. "I don't want all of Adam's fourth-grade book reports to be variations on the theme of *The Babe Ruth Story*. I'd like both kids to know about Amelia Earhart and Madame Curie, too."

"Got it," Barbara said, drying her tears. "Examine all literature for male sexism. Will do. How about art and music?"

"Barbara, for God's sake, the man is an Ivy League graduate. Let's give a little credit where credit is due. Just because he played football, it doesn't mean he's a cultural dwarf! Give him a break. Remember when we were in Florence together? Just try to recall who went back for a second round at the Uffizi and who went shopping for bargains in gold jewelry, huh?"

"Forgive me, I lost my head," she said smiling. "Anything else?"

There really wasn't much I could think of, now that we were down to it. Except. . . .

"Oh, damn, this is so petty, I'm embarrassed to even mention it," I said.

"We're talking about your children; nothing is too petty. If it matters to you, tell me. Don't make me guess." She said it so beseechingly, I had to tell her.

"Promise not to laugh," I said. I now sounded to myself like the giggling adolescent I'd remembered when beginning this dialogue.

"I promise," she said gravely.

"Okay. Barbara, if I die, I want you to swear to me, right here and now, that you will not allow Neill to choose the children's clothes! Under no circumstances is he to decide what they wear."

"Are you serious?" she asked, trying to stifle her laughter and failing.

"I am, you should excuse the expression, deadly serious! The man has no fashion sense whatsoever! If I find out that my adorable children are walking around like schleppers I will roll over in my grave and point directly at you. Understand? If Neill is left to his own devices I know checks are going to get mixed with stripes, and sneakers will be worn with dark socks. Mark my words! Unless you take over the matter of clothing them, you might as well bury all their Lacoste shirts and Saks Fifth Avenue dress-up shoes with me!"

We laughed until we were rolling on the beds, convulsed by the silliness we were so desperate to embrace. And Neill and Irwin stood in the doorway, staring at us blankly, while we gave ourselves up to the giggles.

"Whatever you two are smoking, would you mind sharing it?" Neill finally said.

"We can't," Barbara said. "But Neill—I love the tie you're wearing."

WE WERE ONLY A FEW BREATHS SHORT OF THE HICCUPS, still sputtering away when Dr. McMurtry knocked politely.

"Sounds like a party," he said amicably. "It sounds good." Neill made the introductions; it was all rather like one of those rare cocktail parties where the host is genuinely proud of his opportunity to bring bright, accomplished, good people together for the first time.

"Your friends can stay if they like," Dr. McMurtry said. "I just wanted to tell you what you can expect tomorrow."

Barbara and Irwin excused themselves quickly, promising to be just down the hall.

Dr. McMurtry began by telling us what we already knew.

"The arteriogram wasn't able to tell us all that we had hoped it would before we do the surgery." Was there sadness in his subdued voice? Disappointment? It was impossible to tell where his slow, patient speech was headed.

"There is one more test we'll be doing very early in the morning. And we're hoping that test will be more helpful in isolating the cause of your hydrocephalus."

Hydrocephalus. Water on, in, around the brain. I could feel it lapping against the shores of my skull. I didn't need Mike Margolin, or Billy Di Mauro, or Melinda Marks to define this word for me.

"What's the test like, Doctor?" I asked, trying to control the waterbound imagery that sloshed across my consciousness.

"We call it an air study," he began. Marvelous, I thought. This whole thing is beginning to shape up like a course in Elizabethan drama. I had Water and Air. Any minute now I expected a fourth-year medical student to cross the threshhold gingerly carting Earth and Fire.

61

"The technical name for it is *pneumoencephalogram*." Aha! That brief visit from Bo Peep had been no nightmare apparition interrupting my catnap, after all. The pneumo, she'd called it. "The pneumo will tell it all." I struggled to remember what else she might have said about it while Dr. McMurtry continued to explain.

"We'll take you up to the operating room about seven o'clock in the morning and place a burr hole in your skull . . ." A hole in my head. First thing in the morning. And some people call their first cup of coffee an eye-opener! The lucky fools!

"Just exactly how do you do that?" I asked against my better judgment.

"With a drill," he said simply.

"I see. With a drill," I said. I looked at Neill. Beneath his early summer suntan he had begun to turn the color of my bedsheets. Dr. McMurtry saw it too, I was sure, but he went on.

"Then, we'll take you from the operating room back down to where you had the arteriogram today, and we'll—"

"You keep saying 'we,' doctor. *We* will do this and *we* will do that. Who is the *we*?"

"Well, I'll be assisted in this procedure and in the shunting by several senior residents in neurosurgery."

"Students," I said, hoping he'd contradict my growing conviction that the surgical invasion of my brain was a laboratory exercise for those still learning. Those still learning by their mistakes, perhaps.

"No, ma'am," he countered vehemently. "These are well-trained, highly skilled doctors who have been doing these procedures for several years."

There must be an addendum to the Hippocratic Oath, I thought, that applies only to teaching hospitals: a professional imperative to defend the rights of the young to learn by experience. The accumulation of knowledge was the overriding concern when weighed against possible harm to the patient—or so it seemed to me.

In the case of the operation to install that precious little tube called a shunt, I knew it for a fact. Hadn't Mike Margolin told me himself that he'd been allowed to assist in a shunting case when he was chief resident in neurology in this very hospital?

How many patients, I wondered, had gladly handed over four-figure fees to famous surgeons who never touched that patient in the operating room? Thousands, I thought. Thousands have blissfully gone to sleep under a general anesthetic believing that the

master was in charge when, in fact, they'd wind up being knifed by the big man's underling. Once the lights went out, who'd know the difference?

"I want *you* to do the drilling," I said as forcefully as I could manage to a man who had given me no real reason to distrust him. "Nobody else. Only you."

"I will," he said. "You have my word."

The "code of the west," I thought. If you can't trust a Texan, who can you trust? I tried to concentrate on Sam Houston and Pecos Bill instead of Lyndon Johnson and John Connally while Dr. McMurtry continued to explain things.

That burr hole would allow air to be introduced through a tube into the ventricle. It was possible, Dr. McMurtry warned, that this procedure might not furnish sufficient information. If that turned out to be the case, there was a way to garner more data on the spot. Another hole, this one in my spine, could be created in the nether regions of Diagnostic Radiology as I sat in a chair.

"But we'll only do that if we're unable to see a blockage in the first pictures," Dr. McMurtry assured me. But I was not reassured. I understood the danger intuitively before he had finished his explanation. To me the procedure sounded just like an air compressor attached to a jackhammer—but unlike concrete, my brain was not to be blown apart, only photographed.

"It sounds awfully risky, Jim," I heard Neill venture. (When had he begun to call Dr. McMurtry "Jim," and why couldn't I?)

"Well, we try to minimize those risks as much as possible by proceeding with extreme caution."

Risks. Extreme caution. Particularly terrifying words coming from a man who'd been so otherwise comforting in his diction.

I asked it straight: "Is this test more dangerous than the surgery itself?"

He shuffled his feet for a few seconds and stared at the floor. "Well," he said, "I wouldn't want to say that . . ."

"You don't have to say it," I told him. And he never did say it to me.

But he said it to Neill. Later, in one of those down-the-hall tête-à-têtes that set my teeth on edge, Dr. McMurtry told Neill that the administration of a pneumoencephalogram was among the most precarious procedures in medicine. In all but a few instances, the pneumo had been made obsolete by the CAT scan. Mine was one of those instances, Neill told me sadly.

"They could quite literally blow my brains out, couldn't they?" I said to Neill when he brought me the hallway report.

"Yes, they could," he said.

I could hear meal carts being rolled down the hall outside my room. Lunch time? Or was it dinner—where had the day gone?

"You know what, love," I said to Neill. "Why don't you round up Barbara and Irwin and go home. The kids will be having dinner soon and even the most energetic grandparents run out of steam eventually."

"Are you sure?" he asked in a dry, hollow voice.

"I'm sure. Go ahead. I'll just read and probably fall asleep again. Go on home and open a bottle of scotch. And pour heavy."

"Jeez, that sounds like a good idea," he said a little too convincingly. But he kissed me hard, handed me a stack of *New Yorker*s, and promised he'd be back in a few hours.

A few seconds later, he stuck his head in the door.

"You're sure you don't want me to stay? The doctor is coming back later tonight; I'd hate to miss him."

"I'll take notes for you if you're not here," I said. "Now beat it, partner!"

He was gone. I got out of bed and closed the door against the clatter in the hall.

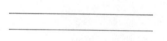

"Just you and me, kid," I said to my brain when we were finally alone together. "What do you want to do tonight?" I climbed into the skeletal bed and looked out the grimy window.

Come on, I said to the brain that was myself, you're supposed to be such a fine specimen, such an inventive organ. Why don't you tell me a story? A cozy, little bedtime story. Something that will entertain me, amuse me. Take my mind off my mind.

A little Dorothy Parker would be nice about now. Something witty and light. Can you do me a few turns of "The Waltz?" That would be perfect.

Once, during a long-ago interview for a copywriting job at a major advertising agency, the man questioning me had said something that stuck. After examining my portfolio, he had asked me a number of cute questions, designed to test my ability to think on my feet. When the questions stopped, he looked me dead in the eye and announced, "You, my dear, have a fertile brain." I was twenty-five at the time.

Fertile. Inventive. Potent. Resourceful. I'd heard all those words and more said about my brain.

"Brain," I whispered to the empty room, "I'd be lost without you." And I fell asleep, dreaming about the Wizard of Oz.

I woke up understanding my dream completely. Just you think for a moment of all those innocents tripping down the yellow brick road, and ask yourself: who among them has *really* got a problem?

You can immediately dismiss the case of the Cowardly Lion. He'll get by on looks alone. Dorothy and Toto? Well, at least they have each other. And besides, most of the kids I know who grew up in Kansas spent their time trying to figure out ways to get *out* of Kansas. So much for Dorothy's credibility.

That leaves the Tin Woodsman and the Scarecrow. And it would be a stiff race, I admit, if the Tin Man weren't so adorable to begin with. Even without one, the guy is all heart. So that leaves you-know-who belting out "If I Only Had a Brain" to the wide-eyed Judy Garland.

And if there's any justice at all in the Land of Oz, his case gets first priority. "If I only had a brain," the Scarecrow sighs, "I could think . . . I could ask questions . . . I could learn!" Not a bad summation for a scarecrow, I was thinking as Dr. McMurtry knocked.

"Come on in, Doctor," I said. "I was just telling myself a story."

"A good one I hope," he said. "Is it one you wrote?"

"No," I said truthfully, "but it's one I'm beginning to appreciate more and more. Would you answer a question for me?"

"If I can," he said, sitting down on the bed opposite me. Where was his retinue, I wondered. Why was it that he, unlike Melinda Marks and all of the other specialists who'd paraded through my door all day, kept coming in alone?

"How is it that you manage to travel all by yourself, Dr. McMurtry? Everyone else seems to be followed by a procession of students, but you keep arriving solo."

He smiled, a bit shyly, and explained that Neill had asked him to keep everybody else out; that I was wary of my guinea pig status.

I was incredulous.

"And you're willing to honor that request?"

"As much as I can," he said. "Any other questions?"

Why be coy, I thought, go ahead. If you can't ask questions, what's a good brain for, anyway?

"Tell me about the possibility of a brain tumor," I said. "I think I understand the other diagnosis, aqueductal stenosis, and what that would mean for me, but nobody has even given the possibility of a tumor a name."

"Pinealoma," he said too soon, "meaning a tumor of the pineal gland."

Pinealoma, I repeated to myself. "Well, if you're going to have an exotic tumor, it might as well speak to you of Hawaii and mai-tais," I said with false gaiety. Bring on the grass skirts.

"Actually, they've had very good results with pinealomas," Dr. McMurtry said evenly.

"Who is *they*?" I wanted to know.

"Radiologists. Therapeutic radiologists." It was the first mention of radiation. This good man was full of ugly, understated surprises.

"You mean if I had to choose a brain tumor, I could do worse than pick myself a pinealoma?"

"A lot worse," Dr. McMurtry nodded.

I could not keep myself from asking what seemed to be the obvious question: "If it's such a fine kind of tumor, Doctor, why don't you just cut it out when you're in there installing the shunt tomorrow?"

"Because we can't reach it without doing damage," he said simply.

What did "damage" mean, I wondered, but decided not to ask. A healthy brain asks a lot of questions, it's true. But a healthy brain also tells you which questions *not* to ask.

A TINY BALD MAN IN A WHITE TUNIC CAME TO SHAVE MY HEAD. He carried a white metal basin and a small, rectangular case made of worn leather.

"I'ma gonna give you the haircut, missy," he said brightly. "My name is Salvatore. But like it says here," he pointed to the bright blue plastic name tag pinned to his concave chest, "you could just call me 'Sal'."

Why, I thought to myself, would anyone on such a grisly mission want to identify himself so clearly? Does the hangman paste a name tag on his black hood that says "Hi! I'm Ralph!"?

With his crinkled grin and his affable manner, Sal should have been doing light trims in a three-chair barbershop in Queens. What in God's name was he doing here?

"Do you like your work, Sal?" I asked him. I was stalling. He knew it and I knew it. He shrugged and lost his grin.

"I try the best, missy," he said with all the resolution one could hope for in a man of his macabre calling.

I asked him if I could go to the bathroom before he began.

"Why not?" he said. "You gonna throw up?"

"No. I just have to go to the bathroom," I said with forced dignity. "Do a lot of people get sick over this?"

"Some. Mostly the ladies."

I crossed the hall to the small bathroom provided for patients whose sparse accommodations did not include private facilities. I didn't need the toilet; I needed the large mirror. I was not about to suffer this parting in public; if I was going to be without my hair for however long this heinous journey lasted, I wanted a private farewell.

I stood in front of the mirror and ran my hands through my hair like a lover. I piled all its chestnut thickness on top of my head and watched my eyes brim. I pulled it hard away from my face and began to braid it. I pulled apart the braid and made a French twist.

Oh, God, I said to the long-haired woman in the cloudy mirror, I'll miss you. Hurry back!

Across the hall, Sal was humming "Volare," tapping his foot to his own rhythms.

"You ready now, missy?" I will never be ready, I wanted to say to him. Knock off the rhetorical questions.

A straight-backed wooden chair had materialized in my cell; Sal motioned for me to sit down.

I stared intently at the silvery razor and white basin that lay on the bed, like a child who cringes at the sight of the needle that will innoculate her but cannot bear to look away for fear she will be pricked unexpectedly.

Something touched my head and I flinched, goose bumps rising on my skin. What was he doing? He seemed to be dividing my long, heavy hair into sections and pinning the coiled sections against my head, exactly as it is done in beauty salons all over the world. Perhaps Sal had a different history than I'd imagined. Maybe he belonged at Sassoon, not Tony's in Queens.

"Is this the way you do it for all of the brain surgery patients?" I asked him.

"No, missy. Only when they got so much hair, like you." Again, just like at the hairdresser's, I couldn't tell if that was meant to be a compliment or a complaint.

I'll bet he doesn't do it for everyone, I thought as he finally began to snip. I'll bet he doesn't do it for the ones who arrive by ambulance and go directly to surgery. The breathless, clock-ticking emergencies, surely they didn't get this meticulous service.

I remembered what Barbara, already the mother of two when I gave birth to Adam, had said when I complained about the pre-delivery shave between my legs: "You dummy," she'd laughed. "You went in too *soon*! The trick is to sit in the car or stand in the hospital parking lot until you can't hold out another second, and *then* get admitted. That way, there's no time for anything except catching the kid on the fly!"

Ah, Barbara! The trouble is you never met Salvatore.

"Well, missy, that's it," he said, startling me out of my hirsute reverie. "How you like it?" That infectious grin had reappeared, wrinkling his scalp.

"So fast?" I said, reaching to touch my forehead with trembling fingers. My fingers felt hair! I clapped my hands against the sides

68

of my head. *Hair!* Behind my ears . . . hair! The crown . . . hair! No doubt about it! Only when I reached to the base of my skull did I discover the skinned surface of my scalp. It was too good to be true.

"That's all? You're finished? No more?"

"That's the whole job," he chimed, fairly bursting with good will. "Your Dr. McMurtry give me strict instructions. Now, how you like it?"

I raced across the hall to the bathroom mirror; from the front, from the sides, and from as far as I could see by twisting my neck, I looked exactly as I had before. I could have auditioned for the road company of *Hair.*

"I love it, Sal!" I shouted across the hall. "You do great work!"

He was packing up his tools when I came bouncing back into the room, humming the same tune he'd begun when he first entered.

"Well, missy," he said, extending his soft hand, "good-bye and good luck."

My spirits soared. "Thank you, God," I breathed aloud. Maybe it had been just a lucky roll, and a trivial one at that. But by now I was taking nothing, *NOTHING* for granted. Whatever little breaks were coming my way, I promised God I'd be punching them in. My big score card, the one that had a space for every day of my life, was a lace doily, it was so full of punched holes. And before today, I'd been using it to wipe my nose; how blind I'd been to its value!

When I'd finished my informal prayer, there was a surplus of gladness that needed to be shared. I dialed my home.

"Mommy!" Adam squealed, when he recognized my voice, "guess what we're having for dessert?"

"Did Grandma Lucille bake her famous mandel bread?" Those crunchy raisin-filled cookies were my mother's favorite curtsey to her Jewish-grandmother role.

"No, no!" Adam declared gleefully, "something much, much better! Guess again, Mommy."

"I give up, Adam. What is it?" My innocently artful son paused dramatically, and then whooped "Hot! Fudge! Sundaes! With whipped cream, Mommy!"

"Adam," I said, "you are some lucky kid. It sounds like you're having a swell party. Can I talk to Todd?" There was that babble of exuberant children's voices that is confusing when you are with them, and totally incomprehensible over the telephone. When it ceased, Adam candidly informed me that Todd preferred to stay with his hot fudge rather than speak to his Moomie.

"That's okay," I said, lying through my teeth and wishing someone would show up with a hot fudge sundae for me right about now. "Let me talk to Grandma, honey."

"She's not here. She's at the hospital. Wait a minute. Do you want to talk to Grandpa Bert? He's baby-sitting us. . . ." My father's voice took over, an odd blend of tension and hot fudge indulgence. Only for him was this call difficult.

"Hi, Dad," I said, trying to picture my thick-skinned father yukking it up with a couple of chocolate-covered kids while his own firstborn was rockbound just a few miles down the river. "It sounds like you're doing a masterful job of holding down the fort there." It was my best try at lightheartedness.

"Yup." To beat my father at laconic you have to reach all the way back to *High Noon*. Only Gary Cooper could do it better.

"I take it Mother's on her way to the hospital?"

"Yup. She should be there any minute. They all left about ten minutes ago—Barbara, Irwin, Neill, and your mother."

Your mother, he'd said.

To her face, he always called her "dear." She hated the name Lucille, and she was right; it fit her not at all. My Doris-Day-lookalike mother should have been named Suzanna or Laura, something with a lot more class, a lot more pizazz. So he called her "dear," and beneath that stiff upper lip, he meant it. But to my brother and me, he always said "your mother." As in "don't talk to your mother that way," or "doesn't your mother look especially pretty today?"

"How you doing there, Bop?" he asked. So I was still Bop. A day of ministering to my children had not disturbed that early morning attachment.

"I'm doing fine, Daddy," I said. I told him the story of my happy haircut and segued right into a jolly little discussion of how to clean up hot fudge. I wanted to end this conversation as happily as it had begun.

"Will you be here in the morning?" I asked.

"Wouldn't miss it," he said, trying for nonchalance.

"Bring me some hot fudge, will you? And coffee ice cream?"

"You got it!" I thought that was the end of the call.

"Karen," he said, his voice breaking over the syllables, "I love you." I hung up and held my head in my hands.

What pain I was causing them—my parents. Me, who always brought home the straight "A" report cards and the winsome boy-

70

friends and the crowd-pleaser awards; who had laid the showcase son-in-law and the precious grandchildren at their feet like shiny pebbles on the shore. What pain!

By the time my mother walked through the door I was up to my aching eyeballs in extended self-pity and guilt so thick it filled the room like fog. Ah played harrible.

"Mom," I said, clutching her hands. "I'm so sorry! I'm so fucking sorry to do this to you—"

"Listen, my darling daughter," my mother said sternly. "You have nothing to be sorry about." She took my face in her hands and looked at me as she must have when I was a small child, her face full of a mother's conflicting love and frustration. "If you think for one minute that you won't get through this, you are wrong, Karen!"

Ah, so that's how the game was going to be played. We were going to parlay the power of positive thinking into an all-purpose coping strategy. No wonder she was all gussied up in her powder blue linen pants suit. No wonder she smelled of Replique perfume and her makeup was so perfectly applied. Beware, Neurological Institute! The mother tiger stalks at break of day!

Determined that this evening would not become a gloomy replay of the night before, I suppressed my own instincts to lighten up, and grew silent. Let them carry the ball this quarter; after all, I'd put together a pretty fine lineup. There was my husband, who had scored so well playing "breezy" with Melinda Marks this afternoon. And Barbara, who was into a damn brave monologue about how a husband could be replaced any old time, but just where was she going to place an ad for a best friend, "Experienced. Send résumés."

"I could run it in the *Chicago Tribune*," she mused, "but I'd wind up with a white-haired little Republican lady who mistook 'friend' for companion and was already packing her white gloves and straw hats for the cruise to Bimini."

My mother gently reminded Barbara that her current best friend was, until further notice, a New Yorker. Therefore, she said, continuing the game, perhaps Barbara should consider placing her request in the *New York Times*, or perhaps the *Village Voice*.

71

"Mrs. Osney," Barbara said with the respect that was a holdover from high school, when everyone's mother had been "Mrs." Somebody. "That's a terrific idea, except that the *New York Times* doesn't run personals and the *Village Voice* classifieds have very little use for a request that doesn't even hint at whips and chains."

"That's not true," I said. "And furthermore, don't knock it until you've tried it!"

"Hey, sophisticated lady!" Irwin called in his best mob snarl, "when's the last time you were into S and M?"

"I managed to wind up here, didn't I?" I said, batting my eyelashes.

"She ain't down yet!" my mother cheered.

And that's how it went on the eve of my brainstorm; that's how we all played the game. Nobody walked on eggs, but everyone was light on his feet.

"I wonder," I said, "if while Dr. McMurtry is in there, he couldn't do a small custom installation. Nothing elaborate—just a tiny switch that could cure tone deafness."

"Forget it," Neill said. "What you really need is an inner tennis button. Let's order *that*." Poor man, he could tolerate my singing off-key, but he was fed up with offering me a handicap in a game that was supposed to begin at love/love.

"If it were *my* cerebral plumbing," my mother said, jumping head first into the well of black comedy, "I'd ask him to remove the part that manufactures guilt. Wouldn't it be wonderful to single-handedly devour an entire Sara Lee cheesecake without feeling any pain?"

It was like playing "If I Had Three Wishes." Everyone's choices were unexpected and slightly whimsical. Nobody got down to it. The closest we came to anything authentic was Irwin's suggestion that Barbara could benefit from a hold button that would paralyze her left hand every time it reached for a charge plate—an intriguing proposal from a man who owned five cars.

No one wished for heightened intelligence, I noticed. Perhaps that said something wonderful about this crew of my nearest and dearest, but to me—whose head was going on the block in a matter of hours—it was perplexing. The question that had been tugging at my gut all day finally found a voice.

"You know what?" I ventured against all the makeshift jocularity. "I keep wondering . . . when all of this is over for me . . . will I still be smart?" Silence fell like cold rain. Bodies tensed, eyes looked away.

"I've been meaning to talk to you about that," Irwin said, crashing the hush with the skill of a diamond cutter. "For a long time now, I've felt you had a highly inflated view of your own intelligence!"

Anyone else would have gotten a fast five between the eyes for that crack; Irwin was rewarded by a full-blown case of the hiccups—mine, and everybody else's.

Dr. McMurtry, who I couldn't help but notice had a remarkable sense of timing, entered to find us still gasping with laughter. What must he think, I wondered; perhaps that when he and his coterie of anonymous colleagues were finished working me over, I might benefit from a brief stay at Psychiatric Institute, Neuro's neighbor with bars? Or had he witnessed other such desperate frolics on the night before brain surgery? In the land of the blind . . . and all that?

"I want to thank you for your orders to the man who gave me the haircut," I said. "That was a glorious surprise."

"I'm glad you liked it," he said modestly. And then, with authority, "visiting hours are over, I'm afraid. Karen's got a big day tomorrow. Let's let her get all the rest she can."

It didn't matter; his entrance had presaged their exit, anyway. The shuffling of feet, the jiggling of car keys—all of those subtle gestures that mean "the doctor is here, we gotta beat it fast"— had been displayed from the moment he entered the room. It wasn't just the lateness of the hour.

Why is it that just at the moment when the patient is going to need it most, the precious support system of family and friends can be found scurrying toward the hospital parking lot? What is so magical about the sound of a doctor's voice as he enters your hospital room that, no matter what he's got to say, your visitors hear it as "the party's over?"

Unfortunately, what is left behind when visitors press those elevator buttons and head for the hospital lobby is the one person least able to understand and absorb the often complicated information the doctor is about to deliver. What if he's got good news? The patient has no one with whom to rejoice; and if the report is negative, it echoes off the walls of the empty room like thunder.

"Somebody," I wanted to scream to my husband, my mother, my friends, "just one of you, please! Stay!"

But I didn't scream it, or even whisper it. And nobody stayed.

P LEASE," I SAID, "I'M SO CONFUSED. JUST ONE MORE TIME."

So once again, Dr. McMurtry explained what he hoped the pneumoencephalogram, scheduled for seven o'clock the next morning, was going to accomplish.

As he calmly retraced for me the path that the air pumped into my head would take, how the pictures would look in a normal brain—all of the ventricles and the aqueduct showing up black—I pondered. Whatever diagnosis could be made from this test, the results would change nothing for him. If it were a tumor, he couldn't reach it surgically. If it were aqueductal stenosis, he had already scheduled the shunt surgery to counter that for tomorrow afternoon.

"Tell me again about aqueductal stenosis," I asked, feeling the fool. He'd already told me twice. "You said it's a congenital defect. Does that mean it's in the genes? That it can be inherited?" My God, could my small sons be walking around with it?

"Hey," he said kindly, "somebody told me you were once an English teacher. 'Congenital,' you should remember, means existing at or from birth. You don't have to worry about your children."

"A mind reader from Houston," I laughed. "What do you know!" That had been my only fear of that diagnosis, and I might have lived with it chewing on my heart for weeks had I not asked the question.

"Well, then," I said, "if that's the case, I want all my money on aqueductal stenosis. To win."

"We all do," he said. "But let me remind you that if this turns out to be a pinealoma, they've had fine results with radiation."

They. First there was *we* and now there was *they.* I didn't even know what *they* looked like, the therapeutic radiologists. I pictured pale, expressionless people who looked like characters created by Rod Serling to populate the "Twilight Zone." No doubt they were to be found at some subterranean level of this building, surrounded by walls of lead.

"Fine results," I repeated. "What does that mean, Doctor?" Numbers, I wanted numbers! Percentages! There is nothing like a life-threatening medical trauma to transform a nongambler into Jimmy the Greek.

He wouldn't give me numbers. Not that night. Instead he gave me a sleeping pill, a pat on my precious head, and bade me good night.

It was one of your go-for-broke sleeping pills, not the variety that leaves you tossing and turning, wondering if and when it's going to work. This was strictly lights out. And on that night, I dreamt of the old five-and-dime store on State Street in Chicago.

When I was a child, my mother would pack up my baby brother Rick and me, and take us to the Chicago Theater for what were to be the very last of the live stage shows. Then when the shows were over, when Martin and Lewis had taken their last bows and Frankie Laine had finished the encore of "Mule Train," she would bundle us up in our dress-up coats and, holding tight to each of us by the hand, walk us across State Street to the fairyland that was Woolworth's.

In addition to the glittering array of ribbons for my braids and gaudy costume jewelry for playing grown-up, that store had another, much more alluring feature—demonstrations, live demonstrations. They were stage shows unto themselves: bright lights, a platform, a microphone, and a real live person whose amplified spiel could be heard in every corner of the huge emporium.

Whatever the merchandise being hustled, there was always a spellbound crowd at the foot of the platform. My mother always knew where to look for me if we got separated in the aisles. I'd be standing there, mouth agape and eyes blazing, staring at the man who was attacking a head of lettuce with some marvelous, irregularly shaped tool that could "slice it, dice it, roast it, toast it, shake it, bake it, dye it, fry it."

I dreamt myself back to that store, that demonstration. But in my dream, it wasn't lettuce up there on the chopping block—it was my brain. Dyed. Fried. Roasted. Toasted. Sliced. And diced.

A pneumoencephalogram is the ultimate mind blower; take it from me. Sunshine cast shadows on the walls as I was wheeled to the operating floor; even under sedation I could clearly identify my husband, my mother, my father, and Barbara jogging alongside the cart. This was a bad sign. First of all, the pneumo was supposed to be only the exhibition bout, not the main event. But their faces—their faces looked as though not only was this the main event, but I was being sent in to go fourteen rounds with Muhammad Ali.

In the operating room I could hear what sounded distinctly like Beethoven's "Eroica." I thought I must be dreaming.

"Is that Beethoven?" I heard my own slightly dazed voice ask, as I lay face down on a table that had a hole for my head to fit through. I stared directly at the floor and focused on feet covered with surgical green.

"Yes, it is," a voice I didn't recognize answered promptly.

"Dr. McMurtry? Where are you?"

"Right here, Karen. Try to relax. Listen to the music. We're about ready to start." It was definitely his voice I heard through the swells of music. Why wasn't I asleep? They were standing there, all of them in their green booties, about to drill holes in my head, and I was awake! In all of my urgent questioning, my intense yearning to be a well-informed patient, I had neglected to confront the matter of consciousness. Why wasn't I out cold, or at least more sedated?

"Will I be able to hear the sound of the drill?" I asked, with total coherence.

"Yes, ma'am." It was unquestionably Dr. McMurtry's voice. "But you won't feel any pain. Just the vibration."

And then they were at it. Drilling through the back of my skull with a sound exactly like a jackhammer boring its way through concrete. A detonation began in my brain and reverberated against the roof of my mouth like an earthquake snaking its way along the fault line of my body. Suddenly, the room was still.

"Hang on now, Karen. Just once more and we'll be finished." Beethoven had become Rachmaninoff. I could see their feet tap beneath my face.

"Is it all right if I keep my eyes open?" I fully expected to see the drill bit dangling in front of my nose.

"Close them," a faceless voice said.

When I opened them again, there was only the music and the tremor still left in my belly; the drill was silent.

The surgical stage of the pneumo was complete; I was wheeled out of surgery and into the elevator that took me to Radiology.

I lay in the same hallway in which I'd waited for the arteriogram. Somehow they had turned me over, face up, and I knew the place. Neill leaned over me with a clipboard full of white papers, while Dr. McMurtry stood a few paces down the hall conferring with several men in white coats.

"You've got to sign this, Kare," Neill said, handing me the clipboard with a trembling hand. On each of his long, thick fingers he was wearing one of my rings. On his thumb he wore the amethyst and pearl heart he'd given me when Adam was born. On his index finger, the blue enamel and gold ring we'd bought in Amsterdam was jammed against his hairy knuckle.

My wide, gold wedding band (inscribed "with world enough and time") was jammed as far down his third finger as it could be made to go. He had moved his own wedding band to his right hand, and from his wrist dangled the gold mezuzah Jack's wife, Linda, had given me two nights ago.

"You look like a hairy gypsy queen in drag," I told him. "Where did you get all that stuff?"

"You asked me to wear it, don't you remember? When they came to get you this morning, you had to take off all of your lucky jewelry, and you asked me to wear it."

I couldn't remember, but I knew it had to be true. If I had to be separated from all those amulets, the next best thing was to have Neill walking around dripping jeweled protection. Barbara and Irwin's children didn't call me Aunt Carmelita for nothing.

"What am I signing here?" I asked, musing on the fact that I must be more whacked out than I had realized in the operating room.

"The usual," he said. But his hands shook around the pen.

"Don't tell me the usual, buddy. This ain't the usual. We both know that. This one could really do it to me. Read me what it says there. Please."

"Just sign it, Karen. There are no more choices." He handed me a small ball-point pen and I scratched my name across the release form. I thumbed through the pages.

"That's a mighty long form for a simple bread-and-butter procedure, don't you think?"

"That one was for the part of the pneumo that's about to begin. This one," he said, handing me a single sheet of white paper, "is for the shunting surgery."

It's best to give you the pneumo straight—the way Socrates took the hemlock. The patient is strapped into a metal chair with webbed bindings not unlike seat belts on airplanes. Except that if you ever found yourself in an airplane seat with as many safety belts as that chair had, you would cash in your ticket at once and take Amtrack. Or Greyhound even. The patient sits crowned with a see-through helmet that immobilizes the head. Openings in the helmet allow needles and tubes to be passed into the brain. You could locate a mighty satisfactory facsimile of this chair in any state where the death penalty is discharged electrically.

There are, of course, significant differences. The electric chair is a quick, clean one-shot. A pneumoencephalogram can take anywhere from one to four hours; mine took three and a half.

What's more, once you're wired for electrocution, you don't go anywhere. You don't travel during a pneumo either, but the chair you're sitting in has some dazzling moves. In order to get X-ray pictures from all the angles, you and the chair get turned around and around—very slowly. That doesn't mean just horizontally; it's more than just a profile shot those folks at the control panel are aiming for. When I say all the angles, I mean *all* the angles!

The patient is revolved—vertically. It's that dandy little feature that takes the experience out of the category of minor torture and puts it right up there with your basic bed of nails.

As my head rolled toward the floor and air exploded in my brain like dynamite, a voice in me said defiantly, "The CAT scan has replaced this torment! Stop it! Let me have another crack at the scanner."

What a foolish woman! No one builds a hospital that looks like a medieval fortress and then holds a garage sale to unload the contents of the main torture chamber!

From time to time, someone would appear from behind the glass panel where the controls were and tell me I was doing fine. I supposed that meant I hadn't yet screamed aloud. Or called anyone a barbarian.

Tubes blowing air in my head, a needle in my spine, hanging upside down like the first car in a roller coaster about to leap the track—that's how fine I was doing. Yeah, sure, just fine.

"She did great," I heard Dr. Marks say to Neill as I opened my eyes, finally back in my room. "I've been getting compliments about her all over the place."

"She was remarkable," Dr. McMurtry intoned. "She really was." I tried to listen, knowing how important a conversation this would soon become. It was all well and good to hear that I was number one on the "martyr hit parade," but there was heavy stuff about to come down and I forced myself to initiate it.

"What did it show, Doctor?" I asked. My voice came out a whisper.

"Well, we'll have to wait for Dr. Lissal to interpret the films. You get some rest now, before we take you back up to surgery to put in the shunt."

"When . . . Dr. Lissal?" I breathed. I could feel sedation around me like a cocoon.

"It will be a while, I'm afraid. He's out of the country."

"Where?"

"Paris."

When the lights went out on me in surgery, I floated across a sea of *mousse au chocolat*.

I WOKE UP IN THE INTENSIVE CARE UNIT; THAT'S THE PART I GOT RIGHT. The part I got wrong was the timing—it was the middle of the night.

"Neill . . ." I rasped. My throat was scraped raw from anesthesia tubes.

"Oh, he'll be along, honey. Now tell me your name like a good girl." A nurse?

"Karen—"

"Say it louder, honey. Come on."

"Karen."

"That's fine, Karen. Now open your eyes . . . uh-uh. Keep them open. Keep them open, Karen! Come on now!"

"What time is it?"

"One o'clock Karen. Now open those eyes for me."

"Day or night?" God, it hurt to talk.

"One in the morning."

I opened my eyes: the window next to my bed was full of black sky. I closed my eyes again.

"Don't do that, honey. Keep them open, Karen!" My voice grated against the nurse's honey-glazed commands.

"I . . . want Neill!" I felt the slippery glass of a thermometer jammed between my parched lips.

Visiting hours in the ICU were twice a day for ten minutes each session—I remembered that from Todd. I remembered! I could remember! The first visit was at 10 A.M.

If it was one o'clock in the morning . . . and the first visiting time was at ten . . . then . . . nine hours. It would be nine hours until I could see Neill. I spit out the thermometer.

"I can do it! I can think!" I cried out. For a split second, I had glimpsed the yellow brick road.

"Thatta girl!" said the pretty Hispanic nurse, retrieving the thermometer and turning to the electrocardiogram monitor of the patient in the next bed.

Ah, yes. The Intensive Care Unit—it all came back to me. I'd forgotten that the ICU was the stainless steel command module on every top-level postoperative mission. A huge room with a high ceiling, decorated wall to wall in varying hues of medical technology. Only Walter Cronkite's studio on election night has more monitors.

But Walter's monitors are there to tell you who won; the equipment in an ICU is designed to showcase the losers. When a patient dies in Intensive Care, the news is bleeped, hummed, and flashed in colored lights. It's a long way from show business, but it is business. Business as usual.

Twice that night I heard the unmistakable sounds of a mechanical epitaph. Apart from that, it was a long and silent night.

I begged for and was refused: a glass of water (no liquids this soon after surgery); a pillow (no elevation of the head for several days—the brain may move inside the skull and cause bleeding); toothpaste (out of the question!); and to be turned over (too difficult with all the wires and tubes attached to my body).

Like most patients in such straits, I wasn't aware of catheters or intravenous needles until they were pointed out to me; but once I knew they were there, I did nothing but complain about them. Why did I need a catheter if I wasn't even allowed to suck an ice cube?

Never mind, I told myself through the unending hours until daybreak. It's over. That's all that matters. It's over.

With the first rays of the sun beating against the window, there came an apparition.

"Mrs. Brownstein," the incredulous voice of the apparition said to me. "What are *you* doing here?"

I opened my eyes to the blessed sight of Dr. Lester Mount's elegant smile. Apollo himself could not have been a more welcome harbinger of a new day.

"Oh, Dr. Mount," I said, "I wanted it to be you who did it!" I struggled to remember the joke about our having a family neurosurgeon, and having found it, decided it was not worth repeating.

"Dr. McMurtry told me that. But you're in wonderful hands and you're going to be just fine." His eyes twinkled and he squeezed my hand—the one without the intravenous needle.

I slept then, until Neill woke me with a kiss.

"Prince What's-His-Name, I presume?" I said when I awakened. Neill took a deep breath and let the tears fall right into his black mustache.

I slept again until it was time for the evening visits. This time I was able to really focus on that clock, ticking away my precious ten minutes. This time I asked about the children, kissed everyone, and initiated my plan to sabotage the command module.

I motioned Barbara to my bedside and whispered conspiratorially, "Bring me toothpaste!"

"Are you nuts?" Barbara chortled. "You're not supposed to have anything in your mouth. Besides, you asked me that this morning."

"Barbara," I said with utter seriousness, "if you are half the friend you claim to be, you will bring me toothpaste. The entire Russian army has just marched through my mouth in boots left over from the 1917 revolution. Now, get me the damn toothpaste or I sign up with the little old Republican lady from the *Tribune*!" The ten minutes were up. They all left smiling.

The next morning's visit brought me something much more wonderful than a tube of Crest—two male aides lifted me up, tubes and all, put me on a cart, and wheeled me out of Intensive Care.

Irwin whispered to me as we rolled toward the elevator, "You're not going back to the old room. Your husband pulled strings. You're getting the top of the line, Mama. Be sure to thank him."

It was a good thing I was forewarned. Under ordinary circumstances I'd have taken one supine glance at my new accommodations and heaved.

I thanked Neill with as much enthusiasm as I could dummy up for the occasion, and when he was out of earshot I muttered to Irwin with bewilderment, "For *this* he pulled strings?"

This was a single-bedded room, smaller than the first. What it had to recommend it, I presumed, was that there were two windows that faced the world instead of mirroring the hospital. Also, with only one bed there, the threat of an incompatible roommate had been destroyed. And there was, to do it justice, a pockmarked porcelain sink in the far corner of the room. Atop the sink sat a fat red and white tube of toothpaste.

"I love it," I said to everyone. "It's gorgeous. Look! There's even a fan on the wall."

Actually, there were two fans on the wall. Two small, black, four-bladed fans, vintage World War II. Identical twins but for the fact that one was hung at an angle to and about six inches above the other.

Dr. McMurtry had warned me about double vision following the surgery. I raised my intravenously appendaged hand and covered my right eye; the top fan disappeared!

"Do you have a headache?" my mother asked carefully when she saw me cover my eye.

"No, oh no," I said at once, trying to reassure her and everyone else whose breath had been held until I'd answered. And then I shouted it. "No! No! I do not have a headache!" They all whooped and cheered and wore me out.

For the rest of that day I slept; it was too soon for anything else. Too soon to raise my head, too soon for even a bedpan. From time to time I'd blink myself awake long enough to use my Grandma-bred politeness in behalf of trying to get an ice chip. Depending on who was on guard duty at the moment of my request, the refusals varied.

"Not yet, honey," was Neill.

"Sorry, Kare," was Barbara.

"No way, Mama." It was Irwin.

"I wish I could, Bop," was my father.

"Not yet, sweetheart, but soon," was Grandma's daughter. The flies returned and did a lot of picnicking with their ophthalmoscopes, but this time they buzzed with reassurance instead of awe. "Extraordinary . . . less than seventy-two hours after surgery . . . did you see her before . . . amazing." It was all a very soothing lullaby.

What wasn't soothing, reassuring, or even worthy of politeness was the across-the-board refusal to answer my sleepy, disjointed questions about diagnosis. It was a simple enough question, I thought, regardless of how inarticulately I was phrasing it: do I or do I not have a brain tumor? All of the answers from all of the doctors were variations on the theme of "when Dr. Lissal comes back and looks at the films. . . ."

"I'll bet he looks a lot like Pauline Kael," I said to Dr. Marks in a moment of bitchy lucidity. "What's the matter with all of you?

Surely you have opinions. Is there a tumor growing in my head or isn't there?"

"Not until . . ."

"When Dr. Lissal . . ."

"We can't answer that . . ."

"You just rest . . ."

If I'd become Jimmy the Greek, the white coats had become the classiest bunch of bet-hedgers since the 1919 World Series.

My family was no help either. For a while, late that afternoon, I was visited by the Suspicion Demons again. They'd come, unbidden, to make a case for "they all know, but won't tell you."

When I finally broke down and revealed my fears, my mother cried as though she'd been wounded. "Oh, Karen, how can you even imagine such a thing, baby? Don't you think we're as anxious as you are to find out?" Those maternal tears and her long-suffering "where did I go wrong?" tone convinced me that they were as ignorant of my fate as I was. But, at least for now, they suffered more for their ignorance than I did.

I slept; they were wakeful, watchful, vigilant. I began to think that the appearance of the twitchy grin Neill was developing corresponded in time with the New York arrival of every single Air France flight.

The way to gauge their anxiety, I thought perversely, delighted with my own skulduggery, was the children. If they're walking in every night and facing children they suspect will soon be motherless, no matter how brave a show they put on, the boys would intuit their torment immediately.

"I want to call the kids," I said to Neill as he was leaving for the night. The private duty nurse had arrived and was hovering solicitously.

"Sure," he said, with what I read as an excess of accommodation. "Todd will be asleep by now, but Adam will be thrilled. When you were in Intensive Care, he kept asking when you'd call." He dialed the phone and put the receiver in my hand.

"Hello?" It was Adam, full of a six-year-old's enthusiasm.

"Hi, Adam."

"Mommy? Is that you, Mommy?" As though I were the one across the Atlantic, not the mysterious Dr. Lissal.

"Yes, dearheart, it's me."

"Oh, Mommy," Adam said at once. "I'm so glad you're better!" Adam is a fairly typical firstborn—a crowd pleaser. Was this his ultimate attempt to please his mother or the real thing?

84

"Who told you I was better, Adam?"

"Everybody. Aren't you?"

"Yes, sugar, I am better," I said, blowing Neill a good-bye kiss and waving my own fifty-dollar-a-night baby-sitter into my room— both of her.

THE PRIVATE DUTY NURSES CAME AND WENT FOR THE NEXT THIRTY-SIX HOURS. Of all of them, only one was able to penetrate the haze of residual anesthesia: a southern-bred widow named Valentine.

With her exaggerated cupid's bow mouth and her hair dyed a shade of red just this side of Hallmark and well past Lady Clairol, Valentine was an exemplary case of "physiognomy is destiny." It wasn't hard to imagine her parents, sixty years earlier, cooing over their baby girl as they'd christened her. "Why, Daddy," her mother must have mewed, "that's just the only name that fits her!"

Valentine had grown into the part. Although her lace edges had frayed and her crimson pucker curved mostly downward, the woman remained a bona fide romantic. Again and again she explained to me that nursing was not work; it was "ministering." You could hear Vivien Leigh's petticoats rustling as she passed among the wounded.

Valentine's chief function, it seemed to me, was to keep my bed-sheets in perfect order. I cautiously searched the bed for a comfortable position, one that wouldn't strangle me in my own tubes or impale me on the intravenous needle. No sooner would I arrange my body in that valuable space than Valentine would come to tug and pat it away.

"I'm just trying to keep you nice and cozy, dear," she'd say, tucking a blanket around my shoulders.

"Valentine," I'd sigh, "there's a heat wave in New York City. It's ninety-seven degrees outside. Forget the damn blanket, please! Instead, why don't you see if you can get someone to fix the fan?" The aged fan had developed a senile buzz that replicated the sound of my skull being drilled, a sound that set my teeth on edge.

"Now, now," she'd say, her voice the sugar cube in a julep, "I wouldn't want one of my babies to catch a chill."

We had very little to talk about, Valentine and I. I slept most of the night; she did crewel work.

In the morning I awoke to find her applying fresh lipstick, using a small retractable brush. Clara Bow lives, I thought, kicking off the covers.

"Our doctor will be here soon," she fairly sang as she smoothed her scarlet coiffure. "Time to tidy up." I knew me and my sheets were in for it but good. She was interrupted by "our doctor" himself. With enormous self-restraint, Valentine managed not to curtsey.

This time Dr. McMurtry was not alone; beside him stood a handsome young man with dark blond hair and weary blue eyes. A resident, I thought; you can always tell. Their eyes are the give-away.

"Good morning," Dr. McMurtry's own eyes looked clear and ready for anything he might encounter in the operating room today. "This is Dr. Harris, chief resident in neurosurgery. He assisted me during your operation."

"How do you do, Mrs. Brownstein," Dr. Harris said, extending his hand. Utterly poised, self assured, and seemingly oblivious to my perturbation with teaching hospital procedures, he sat down on the edge of my bed and began to unplug me. Catheter . . . out. Intravenous needle . . . out. A woman being freed from bondage does not stop to ask her liberator for his credentials—particularly not when he so closely resembles the Richard Chamberlain edition of Doctor Kildare. Instead, she blinks, smiles, and says, "Thank you, Dr. Harris."

Detached from all of the postsurgical apparatus, my senses were free to reassert themselves; I began to reconnect with the world around me.

"I smell breakfast," I said, suddenly ravenous. Somewhere in this formidable stone building oranges were being squeezed, bacon was frying. . . .

"Not quite yet, Karen," Dr. McMurtry said gently. "We'll get you started on some liquids, though, and by tomorrow you'll be ready for a real meal." Valentine tucked and folded with the zeal of a West Point cadet while both doctors admired the floral arrangements that had begun to arrive.

"You certainly have a lot of admirers," Dr. Harris said, sniffing a mass of pale yellow roses.

"Well, she's a very admirable young woman," Dr. McMurtry said as he prepared to leave. Valentine stood at the sink nodding, waiting to be noticed. I remembered Betsy, nodding almost rhythmically to the sound of Dr. Mark's voice.

That must be it, I thought. The repeated nod is the genuflection of doctor worship. I was seized by a fierce desire to smash idols. For Valentine, for me, for all of us who, through a curious admixture of awe and intimidation, distance ourselves from the very people we trust with our lives and possible deaths. Admirable, huh? What was so admirable about me, anyway? Out there, beyond these stone walls, there was no question of definition in my mind: "admirable" meant together, on top of it; the disparate threads of my life woven together—a whole being whose fabric was strong and longwearing.

Here, in this captivity of Lysol fumes, it meant something entirely different: Admirable was docile, accepting, making no waves. Nodding a lot. Like an idiot.

"Admirable, Dr. McMurtry? Oh yeah? Well, how about allowing such an admirable young woman a crack at sitting up? I can't exactly dazzle you guys with my fancy footwork when I'm lying down here!" Valentine flinched as though she'd been bitten by one of the tiny mosquitoes that populated the room.

"Tomorrow," he said, stretching the syllables from Houston to Dallas. "We'll see about it tomorrow." And he and Dr. Harris were gone, the morning sun flashing off their clipboards.

"Well, now," said Valentine, as she stuffed her silk threads and embroidery hoop into a clear plastic shopping bag, "it's time for me to be getting home, dear. You have a nice day, and I'll see you this evening. Take care now."

And so for the next twelve hours I took care, the best way I knew how. I called my children and let them ramble on about who played at which friend's house and who helped Grandma in the supermarket, and what stories the baby-sitter, Janess, was reading to them. I listened to their high-pitched giggles with the concentration I usually reserved for the New York Philharmonic. This composition of shrieking laughter and tinkling giggles had become my symphony.

I let my husband pamper me; sprinkle me with Chanel Number Five dusting powder, life the plastic straw to my lips, smooth my hair.

"You know what that nurse called me?" I said to Neill. "She called me one of her babies. Me! Can you believe it? A total stranger was in here all night just oozing solicitousness. It's no wonder postoperative patients throw up so much. If I'm going to O.D. on tender loving care, I want you to be the pusher, not some fugitive from red dye number two."

Most of the day passed in a sleepy blur of liquids and flowers and pills.

"What are these?" I asked every time a nurse entered with one of those cunning little paper shot glasses.

"Medication," I was told.

"Exactly what kind of medication?"

"Medication ordered by your doctor."

"Which is what?" I demanded with as much propriety as I could summon considering I was seeing two of her and there was only one of me.

"This is for headache," she said, pointing to two clearly identifiable aspirin.

"I don't have a headache," I announced with dignity.

"Yes, but you might. Especially once they start to lift your head this afternoon." I quickly swallowed the aspirin.

"And what's this?" I asked, my hand closing on small hexagonal tablets. These seemed to arrive with the most frequency.

"That's the Decadron."

"What's it for?"

"For shrinking the swelling in the brain after surgery."

"Uh, huh," I said, choking on the water meant to wash them down. "Now, don't tell me," I said, sniffing the minty white liquid in the paper cup she'd handed me. "This must be your nifty little constipation cocktail."

"That's right!" she said with the manufactured brightness that seemed to characterize most of the young nurses on this floor.

They fascinated me, the whole competent lot of them. At the same time these young women were struggling for the gold pins that mark their professional achievement, the women's movement was slapping the hands of little girls who dared to say, "I want to be a nurse when I grow up."

No, no! A thousand times no! You don't really want to be a nurse, sweetheart. You really want to be a doctor. And you *can* be a doctor. And you *will* be a doctor. Now get out there, Allison-Courtney-Jennifer-Melissa-Samantha, and sic 'em! It's a new day.

For some, the gold pins on their caps stuck like daggers. I know because I asked. What was remarkable to me was their willingness to talk about their beleagured profession without seeming threatened by the possibility that a little consciousness raising among the patients might diminish their status. I found it impossible to imagine a senior resident, a man, unburdening himself in quite this way.

"It's sad, really," an especially able nurse said to me one morning. "Those guys are overworked, underpaid, and so locked into role playing that when they take off the surgical masks, they don't even notice they're wearing another mask beneath it." Some new days dawn with muddled colors, I decided.

"Want your television turned on?" the young nurse asked as she folded up the blood pressure kit. "This is a pretty heavy rap for nine A.M. Feel like a little mass media diversion?"

The only media diversion I'd been experiencing at nine in the morning for the last four years was the Muppets of "Sesame Street." And while I had no particular complaint with Kermit the Frog and actually felt genuine fondness for lovable, furry ol' Grover, I was enchanted by the opportunity to escape into more adult fare.

"That would be wonderful," I said. "Could you get channel four? 'Not for Women Only'? You know, the talk show with Barbara Walters?" For a brief spell during Todd's infancy, Adam went to nursery school, Todd slept, and I reveled in fresh-brewed coffee, a quiet house, and Barbara Walters's hard-nosed, perceptive interviews with expert panelists.

"I don't suppose I could have a cup of coffee, could I?" I asked wistfully. The nurse consulted my chart.

"You certainly can," she said. She seemed positively thrilled to be offering so basic a comfort. "And a pillow too, if you'd like."

"Like? Like? Pinch me. I think I died and went to heaven!"

"No, you did not," she said deliberately. "You most certainly did not. How do you take your coffee?"

The day was full of such unexpected pleasures. And one terrible surprise: sometime that afternoon Valentine made an unexpected appearance at my door. She'd gone on a day case when she'd left me, she explained. "Oh, I am weary, my dear," she sighed "Weary, weary, weary. But I just couldn't leave the hospital without bringing you a special treat. I'll be back in a jiffy, dear heart."

What sort of special treat could a woman devoted to the cross-stitch have in mind, I wondered, as she winked and vanished. I played with the possibilities, careful to keep them liquid: a bottomless margarita to cool me against the soaring city temperature; a creamy strawberry milkshake abrim with Nature's own tranquilizer; a root beer freeze from the bodega on Broadway and 166th Street. My mouth had begun to water by the time she reappeared, followed by a tall woman of indeterminate age who was wearing a caftan and a wide-brimmed straw hat.

Oh my God, I thought as I saw the long streamers trailing off the bonnet, she's brought me the ghost of Scarlett O'Hara!

"It's time for me to be getting home, dear," Valentine said as she gave my bed a final proprietary going over. "But I just know you're going to love chatting with Susan here. She's one of my most special patients. You must listen to her now, because you and she, well . . . you've got an awful lot in common now. And she's just about the most inspiring thing I've ever laid eyes on!" She smiled, a row of gleaming dentures piercing the red satin of her lips like an arrow. Then she exited with a self-satisfied "Bye-bye y'all."

Before I had a chance to wonder exactly what Susan and I had in common, Susan took off her hat and flung it on my bed in a gesture so contrived and dramatic that I was forced to look at her. My heart stopped—Susan was bald beneath that hat, bald as a baby's rump.

"Radiation," she said matter-of-factly; and then, from inside the crown of that enormous hat, she drew out two long cotton scarves, one pink and one purple. "Watch this," she said, wrapping her naked head in a whirl of shocking pink.

I did not want to watch this. More than anything on earth, I did not want to watch this. But like the magician who saws the lady in half whether you close your eyes or not, Susan continued to wrap while I continued to feel my heart knock against my chest. I closed my eyes and turned my face to the wall.

"Look," Susan said. "I call this one 'the african turban.' A darling black nurse taught it to me." Slowly, I forced myself to look. Perhaps on a healthy black woman, with wisps of hair peeking through, the elaborate coil of cotton that covered her head might have been attractive. Chic, even. But on Susan, with her pale skin and her demonic blue eyes, it was pathetic. Freakish.

"Sometimes," she said happily, "I wear the hat *over* the scarves." She unwrapped the turban and began to twist the two pieces of cloth around her head while I looked past her.

"What do you think of this one?" she asked, as though I were a rapt audience rather than a terrified witness. "It's on the cover of last month's *Vogue*. You couldn't have chosen a more fashionable time to go bald."

91

"I am not going bald," I said indignantly. "In fact, I can't imagine why that nurse brought you in here in the first place. I think it's marvelous that you've adapted so well to your . . . situation, Susan, but I can't see . . ." I touched my hair, "I simply don't . . ." I grabbed at my hair, "see what any of this has to do with me." I turned my face to the wall again. "Thank you for coming, Susan. Now, please go away."

"I'm sorry," she said as she packed up her hatful of ghoulish tricks. "I was trying to do you a favor. I'm sorry that you weren't ready."

"Ready?" I cried, facing her through defiant tears. "Ready! Susan, I'm not even ready for a lousy bedpan yet, let alone a *Vogue*-inspired glimpse at the future!"

"Look," she said, "I had no idea where you or your head were at when I walked in here. But it's obvious that I came at the wrong time. I'm going home tomorrow. I live in the Village; I'll leave my phone number at the desk. Call me if you need me. For anything."

I didn't thank her. I didn't wish her well. I stared at the wall and wished I had never laid eyes on her.

By THE NEXT DAY I MIGHT HAVE BEEN READY FOR SUSAN . . . ready for anything, in fact. Not only had I taken my first steps down the green hallway, I was itching to fly. High on life, drunk with survival, I floated into my new incarnation: the "born-again princess." Filled with a spirituality bordering on glee, I silently recited every blessing I could remember in Hebrew. I knew full well that some of the prayers were inappropriate and that in my ignorance I was missing others that might have been right on, but it didn't matter. I was a Jew and I had survived. There is no shortage of prayers for that particular combination.

When I had exhausted my limited supply of Hebrew, I switched to English. There was no organ or function of my body for which I did not give thanks. Literally every part of my being was caught up in an appreciation so deep I could feel it swirling through my veins, coursing energy that throbbed through my body. I felt like a highly tuned engine. *This*, I said to myself, *is rebirth*. This is what it means to be given a second chance, a tomorrow.

If tomorrow turned out to be hairless, so what? Screw it! All that mattered was that tomorrow would come.

Still trembling with the joy of survival, I called my house at seven thirty in the morning, woke everyone, and announced I had a full-blown case of "bring me."

Yes, I knew the insidious "bring me" disease was a childish malady not at all becoming to a thirty-two-year-old woman—especially not to one who had spent no little time instructing her own children to avoid it.

"Never mind, Mother," I said blithely, "just get a pencil and write all this down. Bring me:

a picture of Adam and Todd, a recent one
all my makeup
the sabbath service Jack and Linda wrote
my address book
hair ribbons in assorted colors
a Sunday *New York Times*
a notebook and sharp number two pencils
my feathers . . ."

"Your what?" my mother repeated sleepily.

"My *feathers*. Two years ago I got a terrific bargain at a Bonwit Teller lingerie sale: a white silk robe trimmed with ostrich feathers."

"You're kidding," my mother said.

"I am not kidding. I've been saving it for some fantastic man who could convince me I didn't already have the top of the line with Neill." I could hear her sharp intake of breath.

"Which means you'll have to cut the tags off, Mother."

"I'll bring it," she said. "You know you're crazy?"

"I am not crazy—I am reborn!"

"In ostrich feathers?"

"They could have been peacock, Mom. Will you just bring the robe, please?"

"I'll bring it, I'll bring it. Anything else?" My breakfast tray had just been delivered. Stewed prunes and soft-boiled eggs.

"Yes. Two croissants from the bakery on Riverdale Avenue."

"Got it," she said. "I'll be there by ten."

The croissants were only the beginning. I had the most rabid case of the munchies I'd experienced since the first time I'd gotten off on marijuana, and it wasn't just ordinary junk food I was after. Oh, no. I knew exactly what I craved.

I dialed the advertising agency where my friend Jeff wrote some of the most successful and funniest copy in the business; he also served his agencies as in-house food maven. I hadn't seen or heard from him since he'd left my "spirits up" party, although Raniera, his wife (my friend and singles tennis partner), had stayed in close touch.

"Yeah? This is Jeff." This morning he was answering his telephone à la Broderick Crawford.

"Jeff, this is Karen. Bring me prosciutto and melon."

"From Zabar's, right?" he said, as though I were calling from a phone booth instead of Neurological Institute.

"Of course from Zabar's." I said. "And a quarter pound of Brie while you're at it."

"Welcome back, Karen," he said in his own voice. "You'll have it tonight. You want wine?"

"Do I sound like I want wine?"

"No, you sound like you're making your own." I was—my own wine, my own music, my own look-out-world-I'm-coming-through fancy-dress ball.

"Dr. Harris?" I said as I lay flat on the bed while he removed the stitches in my neck where the shunt had been threaded through my jugular, all the while admiring his own handiwork. "Dr. Harris, if it turns out that I do have a brain tumor, and I do have to have radiation therapy . . . will I lose *all* of my hair . . . or just some of it?"

"Karen," he said, laying the tiny bits of surgical thread on a gauze pad, "that's the first dumb question I've heard you ask. That's like saying 'I'm going to a party. Should I wear the blue dress or the pink one?' In your case, all that matters is . . . YOU'RE GOING TO THE PARTY!"

Damn betcha! And in ostrich feathers, no less.

———————————
———————————
———————————

It wasn't just the feathers that made me a born-again princess. It was my attitude—admirable. No doubt about it, I was the Super Patient of Neuro. Princess Admirable.

"You are unbelievable!" Ruth, the Back, whistled as I entered her steamy cubicle around the corner from my own. It had been six days since my surgery, and three of them had broken records for high temperatures. Her room smelled of sweat and alcohol and oil paints.

"Just look at you!" she said, shaking her blue-black head of Gina Lollobrigida curls. "It's a hundred and three degrees outside, you've just had brain surgery, and you're walking around this dump in your sundress and earrings like an advertisement for some kind of luxury cruise. They ought to put you on a poster somewhere—you could be the 'Easter Seal kid of brain tumors.'"

I ignored what I considered to be her premature diagnosis. At least she was able to say the words "brain tumor"; most people, I'd begun to notice more and more, could not. And it wasn't just among the tenderhearted that the words stuck. The very same people who could glide right over "heart attack" and "mastectomy" like licking ice cream off a cone were choking on "brain tumor."

"She has a 'tumor,'" my friends whispered to one another outside my room.

"Were they able to get at 'the tumor'?" they asked Neill, as though it were some unrooted growth, not belonging to my body at all. *Tumor* gave them no trouble; it was *brain* that threw them. And why not? Talk about hitting you where you live! If not there, where?

So no small part of my Princess Admirable attitude was devoted to accepting such reticence with charity and understanding.

Three of my healthy young women friends reluctantly confided that they'd made doctor's appointments since my news had hit them.

"Why?" I asked innocently. "What's happened?" The answers were whispered, embarrassed, shy: "Because I have headaches."

It hurt me that my nightmare had contaminated them, spawned a local epidemic of terror in their otherwise peaceful lives; yet I could not deny them their fear. They too had small children, plans for the future, and, occasionally, they had headaches. If it could happen to me, said a friend I'd played tennis with (and beaten) the day before I saw Melinda Marks, it could happen to anyone.

There was a part of me that wanted to take those frightened people and shake them; shout at them, "You're being ridiculous! Overreacting! Everyone gets headaches. Cancel your appointments. Play tennis instead." And then there was another part of me, the part that remembered being hit from behind, that worried about them and their occasional headaches.

"She got here just under the wire," Dr. McMurtry had divulged to my mother when she'd pressed him. And my mother, struggling to exorcise the Suspicion Demons for both of us, had told me.

"You've apparently inherited your father's high tolerance for pain, Karen." She had said it tonelessly, but I knew by the tears glistening in her eyes that she was remembering my father's massive coronary twelve years before. He had had brief chest pain on a Saturday morning, his doctor had suggested he be hospitalized for surveillance, and, whammo! That night, in the hospital, came the big one.

"You're cut from the same bolt," my mother said stolidly, "you and he. Tough as nails." I let it pass. It was off the mark and we both knew it, but we let it pass. The grim potential of a high pain tolerance could not yet be reckoned with. It was too soon after surgery. Only later, when the first headache might come without explanation, the garden variety headache that you take two aspirin for and forget about, would I be forced into an uneasy truce with my body's cursed disdain for hurting. For now, I was content to float in the pearly delirium of my own survival.

"C'mon, Ruth," I said. "A few of my friends are bringing lunch soon. Let's get someone to move you into the lounge. I've heard an intriguing rumor: there's a slight breeze coming off the river and it can be felt—well, smelled, anyway—in the patient lounge at the end of the hall."

"Naw, you go ahead. My husband's taking the afternoon off and he's bringing lunch."

"Lucky woman. Neill just began back at the office today." Secretly though, I was pleased that Neill had returned to work on however limited a schedule; it was a blessed first step toward normalcy. Short days at the office were better than no days at the office.

"Would you do me a favor, Karen, before you go?" Ruth asked. "Just stay long enough to hold the mirror while I do my face."

So I held the mirror while her artist's hands rendered her lovely face for exhibition.

"You're gorgeous," I said, studying her at close range. "I think you're the most beautiful woman I've ever known."

"Thanks," she said softly. "Now beat it, Brain. Go out there and spread some of that picture-perfect cool around."

Actually, I did feel cool. Intellectually I knew the heat was oppressive; I could see it steaming off the asphalt as I looked out the window, could verify it on the *New York Times* weather page. But physically, physically I felt like a million dollars—in singles.

Like the character in *A Thousand Clowns*, I wanted to shout out the window, "Hey! You out there! Healthy people! I'm one of you!"

I went to my precious little sink and let the mirror confirm what I was feeling. It was true, I did look healthy—better, in fact, than I had looked in months. The same benevolence that had kept me from being scalped had kept me from being turbaned. At the back of my head was a small gauze bandage, easily covered by all of the hair that remained. My skin, perfectly ordinary before the ordeal, was today radiant, smooth, and still tanned to perfection. Even my eyes, which until this moment I had been carefully avoiding, were clear and brighter than usual. The flowers that now seemed to fill every available space in the room framed my face in the mirror.

You know, I said, cracking the Narcissus routine even as I was creating it, you'd better watch it, kid. This whole shebang could wind up being the last rose of summer story. Tomorrow you could die on the vine.

"Up yours, lady!" I snarled at the woman in the mirror. "I ain't no rose! I'm a goddam tiger lily!" And I even managed a reasonable growl before I collapsed on my bed in a heap of exhausted satisfaction.

As on my very first day in the hospital, it was Barbara who woke me.

"Don't get up," she said from the doorway. "Just let me look at you." She had flown home to Chicago once I'd been brought back from Intensive Care; spent three days reassuring her children that her occasional migraines were nothing like Aunt Karen's headaches, and flown back to New York.

"I don't know how you did it, pal," she said, "but when I walked out of here last week you looked like a mock-up for the Bionic Woman. Today I come back and, presto! it's Wonder Woman!"

"Want to see where I hide the magic bracelet?" I said, hugging her and laughing. "It's in the drawer behind the bedpan and the Dermassage."

"Well," she said, removing her smart linen blazer, "however you did it, I'm thrilled. Have they told you when you can go home?" The question stung.

"They don't tell me anything. They bring me pills, and they peek under the bandage, and Dr. McMurtry drawls, 'You're doing fine,' and they don't tell me a goddam thing. Mind you, Barb, I don't ask them much. Occasionally I inquire casually as to whether I have a brain tumor or not, but apart from that I keep my nose pretty clean."

She took it all in, settled back in one of the lounge chairs Neill had borrowed from another room, and said in her Barbara-the-Coper voice, "And? What do they say? You do or you don't?"

I propped myself up on my pillow. "They don't say shit."

"I can't understand. Aren't all of the tests done?"

"Of course all of the tests are done. They were finished looking at my pictures the day I went to surgery."

"Well, then, what's holding them up? What's missing?"

"Ah now, there's the rub. It's not *what's* missing; it's *who's* missing. The head honcho in diagnostic radiology is in Europe, you see, and no one is going to stick his head out on a diagnosis until the Wiz returns."

"And when is that auspicious day?" she asked, innocently.

"Three weeks from now."

"Oh, Jesus," she groaned. "What are you supposed to do in the meantime? Hang by your thumbs?"

"Something like that. I am supposed to go on being everyone's favorite patient, Princess Hang-in-There."

"Don't they even hint? Give a clue?" I knew what question was coming. I had put it to myself often enough when I was alone in the room with that hateful buzzing fan and its ceaseless croaking reminder of what this was all about. When the room was dark and Neill had gone home to crash over a bottle of scotch shared with friends, I would count up the number of times Dr. McMurtry had used the phrase "marvelous results" that day. And then I'd factor in all of the long-distance phone calls from Mike Margolin, who had an open line to Melinda Marks.

"I think I have a brain tumor," I said.

"But you don't *know*," she countered. "You're just guessing, right?" Even the consummate coper slips now and then, I thought, watching the furrow of her brows deepen.

"Cheer up, Barb. You're right. I am just guessing."

"Special delivery from Zabar's!" Raniera announced from the doorway in her mellifluous South African accent. "Where's the lady who ordered prosciutto and melon several days ago?" She and Edye came in, loaded down with shopping bags and daintily wrapped gift boxes.

"Barbara," I said to my friend of long standing, "I want you to meet two special friends of mine, Edye Vogel and Raniera Wolff. These are my children's surrogate mothers." My friends, strangers to one another, embraced in that sober way people of limited acquaintance peck at each other's cheeks at funerals.

When we had devoured the last of the sweet melon and all the jokes about an afternoon blood pressure reading following prosciutto had palled, I asked about my children. It was pointless, I'd decided, to ask either Neill or my parents how Adam and Todd were faring; those opinions were sure to be colored for my benefit. But these women, who were seeing the children every day as they drove them to summer programs they themselves had hastily chosen, would give it to me straight.

"Adam hates his camp," Edye said, as she stood with her back to me, pulling wilted yellow daisies from an elaborate floral arrangement. "But Adam hated day camp last year, too," she added matter-of-factly, "so it's no big deal. And Todd—Todd has become the collage king of his nursery camp. Your younger son has a real flair for pine cones and glue, my dear."

"And," said Raniera quickly, as if they'd rehearsed this duet, "that baby-sitter of yours, Janess, takes them both down to the pool every day after lunch and, all things considered, they are just terrific, Karen."

"The truth, Ren?" I said. Edye, with her wit and her reassuring aura could fool me, but Raniera had eyes as clear as the waters of her homeland, and a porcelain complexion that blushed neon when she was uncomfortable.

"The truth," Raniera said. "Cross my heart and hope to die. And if you've any doubts, just remember what Jeff's always saying about gentiles being such lousy liars."

"Is that your husband?" Barbara asked, reminding me that she and Irwin had put their troubles on hold while I hung by my thumbs. Raniera's eyes clouded.

"My friend Raniera," I said to Barbara, "is a fellow traveler of yours on the bumpy road to love. You have more than just me in common." Barbara gave a stiff little nod; acknowledgment, nothing more. The silence grew awkward, palpable as the heat of midday, suffocating.

"My dear," said Edye, "you need your rest. We'll be on our way." I looked at my watch. Nearly three o'clock—they'd go home, shed their bright summer skirts, throw on bathing suits, and plunge into the swimming pool behind our apartment building. On a day like today it was worth every penny the management of our building charged for it. I felt a quick flash of envy, imagining the icy water on my skin.

"I wish I could dive," I said to Barbara when they'd gone.

"Dive?" she repeated with amused irony. "Aren't you the same girl who had a doctor write a medical excuse for swimming when we were in high school? So you wouldn't get your bubble hairdo wet?" Barbara laughed.

"Yeah, but that was then. This is now." I said.

"You want to learn to dive? I'll teach you the first chance we get, Kare." And she meant it, she who had been the only kid in school with a backyard swimming pool. "When this is all over, we'll all go to Hawaii or Acapulco or somewhere, and we'll dive until your brown eyes turn chlorinated blue."

"I can't," I said, beginning to flirt with the green sea of self-pity and nearly preferring it to the blue waters of the Gulf of Mexico.

"Why not? Do you have a better offer?"

"Nope. I asked the doctors how the shunt would limit my activity and they said there were two things I couldn't do—dive and ride motorcycles." A wave of exhaustion swept over me and I began to laugh and cry simultaneously.

"Oh, boy," said Barbara, rolling her eyes heavenward. "Nap time at the funny farm. I'm going to take off for a while and let you sleep. But before I go, I want to remind you of one thing, lady. In all your life you've never wanted to dive. And as for motorcycle riding, even if I zipped you into one of Irwin's black leather jump-suits and stuck a Dayglo helmet on your priceless head, you wouldn't know a Kawasaki from a Harley Davidson! I'll get you a new pitcher of those ice chips you're becoming addicted to, and then I want you to go to sleep."

"Is that how you talk to your children, Barbara?" I asked, my eyes closing involuntarily.

"Only when they behave like children."

When I opened my eyes it was dinnertime. Neill was sitting in the lounge chair staring at me over the pages of the *Wall Street Journal*.

"Hi, love!" I said, jumping off the bed so fast that there were at least three Neills to hug and kiss. "When did you get here?"

"About an hour ago," he said, cradling me on his lap. "For a lady who could never fall asleep in the daytime, you sure can cut those Z's now." He ran his hands over my body, tickling me at first and then catching my mood, more slowly. "God, you feel good to me," he whispered, his breath warm against my neck. Desire rose in my body like a tidal wave.

"Thank God," I heard my passion speak, "that part still works."

"Did you ever think it wouldn't?" he said, his own voice husky with yearning. I traced the line of his jaw with my fingertips. "No," I said kissing him again and again, sowing us both a field of

101

passion we knew could not be harvested but could not keep from seeding. "But it's lovely to know it for a fact . . . spend the night with me, Neill."

"Here?" he said, dismay releasing his grip on me.

"No," I said, getting up and facing him. "At the Plaza! Of course here, silly. No one will mind; it's a postoperative floor. Relatives of patients sleep here all the time." I looked at the muscles in his thighs, brown against the white of his shorts, and waited.

"Relatives stay overnight because they're worried," he said, "not because they're horny."

"If they ask, tell them you're worried," I said. I saw his dimples work as he considered the proposition.

"I am so worried," he said at last, "I may wet my pants."

S TREAMS OF NERVOUS, DIFFIDENT VISITORS KNOCKED ON MY DOOR over the next few days. They entered cautiously, hiding behind fruit baskets and flowers, their eyes clouded by what they had seen between the elevator and my room.

"Can we come in?" they'd say in hushed voices, peeking timidly around the door.

"Of course!" I'd crow from my high-on-life crest. "The more the merrier!" And they'd enter: the friends, the neighbors, the business associates, wide-eyed at the contrast between what they thought they would find here, and the exulting woman they actually encountered.

Bubbles of relief popped like champagne corks as soon as they saw me. In my feathers and hair ribbons, I'd pass around the fruit, the nuts, and the chocolates and carry on like New Year's Eve in Times Square. And I, to be sure, was a coy Baby New Year, full of innocence and promise.

"You're wonderful," I'd tell them. "You're wonderful to come. You're wonderful to bring me things. You're wonderful!"

And, of course, it worked. "*You're* the one who's wonderful," they would chime. "You're the one who's extraordinary."

I don't remember if I'd coyly bat my eyelashes or look away modestly when they began that chorus of cooing; but I can clearly recall that I did absolutely nothing to discourage it.

The only visitors who refused to stroke me were two who never actually made it to my room: Adam and Todd.

For them, I gave a command performance in the lobby of Neurological Institute. It took me an hour to get ready for their visit. The parties in my room were mere sock hops. This was prom night.

103

"What do you think?" I asked my mother as I arranged my hair over the bandage for the sixth time.

"I think you better get down there before Todd tears the place apart," she said merrily.

"I'm afraid I'll cry," I told her as the elevator doors closed. I hadn't been erect in an elevator here since the day Melinda Marks had escorted me to the CAT scan. "I know I'll cry." The door slid open.

"Mommeeeee!" Todd shrieked, scrambling up my legs into my arms.

"I'm going to eat you, Todd," I said, tasting my tears against his sweet flesh. "I'm going to take bites out of you until there's nothing left . . ." Adam's sturdy little body flew across the lobby and pressed itself against my legs. "And then I'm going to start on your brother," I said as I lowered Todd and scooped up Adam.

"I miss you, Mommy," Adam said in his premature baritone.

"Oh, my darling child," I said, wiping the tears from his bottomless black eyes, "I miss you, too." He wriggled out of my arms, flushed with embarrassment. Strangers were watching.

"I swam under water at camp today," Adam announced. Like the moments following a summer storm, his world could instantaneously revert to sunshine, its natural element.

"I got new shoes, Mommy," Todd chortled, kicking feet that ended in tiny brown leather sandals. "For Calidornia."

"California," Adam corrected with big brother disdain. "When are we moving, Mom?" Adam said suddenly. Was it a throwaway line or a challenge? I couldn't tell. I looked at Neill for help.

"When does Daddy say we're moving, honey?" It was the first time I recalled handing off to Neill since we'd become parents, and it made me feel dizzy to do it now.

"When you're all better." He looked over his shoulder at Neill for confirmation. "Right, Daddy?"

"Right, Adam."

"Well, when will that be?" Adam wanted to know. "When you come home will you be better?" I took a quick peek at how unsettled Adam's world must have become and drew the steel curtain down as fast as I could.

"Not right away, Adam. But soon."

"Well, when?" I had never heard him whine before; the sound scraped against my heart like fingernails on a chalkboard.

"What's the date today?" I asked. Adam paused, figuring it out.

"Um, June. June twenty-fifth," he announced with resolve.

"We'll move before the end of summer," I told him, figuring it out for myself so that all of the bets were covered.

"Promise?" he said, brightening.

"Promise."

Promise . . . California . . . California promise. I lay awake that night and played with the words. They floated, weightless and airy as the sun-drenched lyrics of the sixties. "California Dreamin'," José Feliciano had sung, his head flung back, the notes themselves carrying the promise of the dreams.

California dreamin' . . . bizarre dreams full of tall blond strangers who vanished into a blazing sun when I reached out to touch them . . . enchanted dreams of nut-brown children running barefoot through the foothills. And all of the images, all of the dreams, laced one to another by the morning fog gathered between here and the future. "When I come home to you, San Francisco / Your golden sun will shine / for me."

Sure, it's easy for you to say, Tony Bennett. You're not waiting to find out whether your instructions are to cross the Golden Gate or jump off it. You've got a real edge on me—you can come home to San Francisco; I have to leave home to get there.

"Home," I said aloud to myself. "Home," hoping the sound of the word might point me toward the place. Surely it wasn't three thousand miles across the country, in a rented house.

"It's irresistible," I'd bragged to my friends about Palo Alto. And seeing their faces twist with urban scorn and human envy, I'd amended the boast. "Visually, it's irresistible. Aesthetically, it's irresistible."

"Woman does not live by aesthetics alone," Edye had retorted. "Where are you going to go for theater, my dear? What are you going to do if it rains on a Sunday and there is no Museum of Natural History? What are you going to do when your kids have withdrawal symptoms from heterogeneity because everyone out there is blond and beautiful? What are you going to do then? Huh?"

"Knock it off," I'd say defensively. "Palo Alto is forty-five minutes from San Francisco. It's got Stanford University. Los Angeles is an hour away by plane. The San Diego Zoo is not exactly shabby either . . ."

"Yes, my dear, but what about . . ."

"You? That's what this is about, isn't it, Edye?" She'd covered her face, nodding. "I will visit you at least twice a year, maybe more. Neill will be coming to New York almost as often as he goes to California now. I'll tag along. You'll see. I promise."

Oh yes, I thought, refilling my bedside glass with ice chips. "But I have promises to keep, / And miles to go before I sleep, / And miles to go before I sleep."

Ah, you crafty old poet, you, I thought as I lay in bed sucking on the ice chips. You've got all the answers, haven't you? "Home is the place where, when you have to go there, / they have to take you in."

Robert Frost, the New England poet who wrote "Lilac in me because I am New England, / Because my roots are in it, / Because my leaves are of it, / Because my flowers are for it, / Because it is my country . . ." was born in San Francisco.

"I'm going home tomorrow," I told Ruth, as she lay outside my room. "Back to the warehouse in Riverdale." She took my hand and held it to her face.

"Dammit, Brain," she said, "you're a tough act to follow." Pain crunched against the corners of her mouth. "Call me, will you?"

"I'll do better than that," I said self-consciously, "I'll come and see you."

"The hell you will!" she hissed. "Don't you ever, ever show up in this joint again! Ever!" She licked her lips and, with her arms, pulled the top half of her body up to where she was able to look me right in the eye. "You are free, Karen. Great God Almighty, free! Don't ever look back."

She lay back on the cart, her body heaving with the effort. "I'll call you when I can walk," she said softly. "Expect my call."

TEN DAYS AFTER MELINDA MARKS HAD LOOKED INTO MY EYES and seen something "funny," I came home. It was Saturday, June 26—the day the Brownsteins had been scheduled to move to California. The day the new tenants were to have taken over the lease on our apartment. The day we began to pay rent on the house in Palo Alto.

So much for proper prior planning, I told myself as Neill and I drove north along the Henry Hudson Parkway. So much for long-range goals and preparation. Would I ever again feel secure enough to flip the pages of my calendar and make notations that committed me to the future, bound me to times and places I might never reach?

Perhaps I would have flirted with the cold scenario of a blank future longer if the view hadn't been so splendid. But on the left was the Hudson River, flashing blue beneath the indomitable arch of the George Washington Bridge; and on the right was the summery lushness of the trees that framed the Cloisters. I could not sustain despondency in this setting.

"It's beautiful," I said to Neill. "It's all so beautiful." Neill took my hand and held it as we drove. "It's a perfect day for a homecoming," I said as we approached the bridge. I had fallen newly in love with New York, grateful for the extra days we would have here. California could wait. I could wait.

"I love New York in June," the cornball lyricist in me sang. "How about you?" But instead of extolling Gershwin tunes, as I had expected him to do, Neill was grimacing behind the wheel.

"Oh, I don't know about that," he sighed. "Don't you think the Golden Gate is really more beautiful?" The question was phrased casually, but there was a thickness in his voice that made me ache. I had tripped him in a way I hadn't realized before this moment. It wasn't only the empty house in Palo Alto we were paying rent

107

on, or the fact that the new tenants for our apartment in New York had been bought off when Neill offered to pay their rent as well; those were simple problems: solvable—as Irwin was fond of saying—by throwing money at them.

No, something much more urgent had been held up from the day I was diagnosed—the Neill H. Brownstein Corporation, a new entity that had been nearly three years in the planning. All of the professional dreams and schemes that had convinced Neill that this move to California was right for us were stuck at the starting gate. Where would I find the words with which to make up for this delay in his life?

Here I was, taking New York back to me like a lover I had promised my husband I would never see again, while he pined for the golden west. We passed the George Washington Bridge in silence.

"I don't know, babe," I finally said. "I think it's a stalemate."

"What?" he asked absently.

"The beautiful bridge debate. I mean, the Golden Gate links a city shrouded in fog to Marin—a county that looks for all the answers in the bottom of its hot tubs. Some linkage."

"Yes," he said, catching on, "and the George Washington Bridge links everything with New Jersey. Case closed," he announced smugly.

"Wait a minute, dear," I said as I moved closer to him. "New Jersey is a very cheap shot. Even a woman with holes in her head recognizes a cheap shot when she hears one. You'll have to do better than that."

It was easy to banter this way. Dozens of conversations like this one had filled the years we were living in New York. At bottom was the certain knowledge that we were both city people, wired for city voltage. Chicago. New York. How would the genteel college town that called itself the "City of Palo Alto" be able to support our urban moorings?

Actually, the day we'd moved to New York, six years earlier, we'd known California was the next move. But it wasn't a move right around the corner, whereas Broadway was—and so was Lincoln Center, SoHo, the Plaza, and the Christmas tree at Rockefeller Center. So like tourists on an extended visa, we went and saw and did with the urgency of those who know that this is not forever. Karen and Neill, storing up nuggets of culture and haute cuisine against the possibility of a California drought. It had been a glorious six years.

There were two reasons to give it all up: first and most compel-

108

ling was the fact that Neill was spending nearly a fourth of his time in California anyway. One week out of every month, the three thousand miles of America rose up between us like the Great Wall of China. We built our lives around the regularity of those wrenching separations. Living and working in California was the obvious solution for Neill but I, who had nothing akin to the Neill H. Brownstein Corporation waiting for me there, needed convincing.

So I set about convincing myself. In six trips to California that spanned a period of four years, I looked at the houses, the schools, the career possibilities for women writers, and the endless azure sky. I convinced myself; there was nothing not to like.

"Sounds like damning by faint praise," Edye had murmured suspiciously when I told her we were going.

"Nothing of the sort," I'd retorted. "It's just plain good living out there. And besides, I'm tired of being a single parent every fourth week." Two good reasons.

But now, with the future so clouded that even the perfect skies of Palo Alto appeared menacing, I wasn't so sure. New York, with all its endless mystery, was sanctuary. I had loved that mystery always, delighting in the knowledge that New York could never be exhausted or mastered. There was a delicious security in knowing that its promise was infinite—the totally enigmatic city, I had once called it. How could I explain to self-satisfied Californians how comforting I found that enigma, how dearly I cherished its promise?

"Give it up, sugar," I said, elbowing Neill in the ribs. "Admit it. Some day soon, when you're looking out those monstrous picture windows in your office and all you can see are the Sierra foothills, rolling green pastures, and maybe a few Stanford-educated cows, you're going to long for your old office on Park Avenue. Your pulse will quicken just thinking about making a run to Grand Central for the six-seventeen train." I poked him until he admitted it.

"We'll come back to see the tree at Christmas time," he said softly as we got off the parkway and our building came into view.

"*This* Christmas?" I asked, incredulously.

"*This* Christmas," he said as we pulled into the driveway. The doorman cried when he saw me.

Nothing that had happened to me since I'd left warranted the hero's welcome that greeted me when I came home. The celebration, I knew, was in honor of what hadn't happened to me.

"I am intact," I whispered to Neill as we rode up in the elevator. "We are intact." If my stay at Neuro had diminished me, it had been in ways that were not visible when I got off the elevator on the fourteenth floor that Saturday morning.

As Neill turned the key in the first of three locks, I could hear Adam shouting. "Grandpa Bert! Grandpa Bert! Mommy's home! Now we can move!"

"I have promises to keep," I said to Neill as the door swung open.

"It's a party, Moomie Mommie," Todd gurgled as he pulled me into the living room. "A party for you!" I knelt and he covered me with wet, warm kisses and filled my arms with yellow balloons. This was no warehouse full of cartons; this was the Mormon Tabernacle Choir singing "Home for the Holidays." Adam hugged me hard enough to startle me, and thrust a fist full of crayoned treasures toward me at the same time.

"Well," he said, his eyes shining. "How do you like it?" How do you like your party?"

I looked up at my mother and father. Tears trailed their strained faces as they stood watching, dwarfed beneath a thirty-foot banner that stretched across the living room. "Welcome Back, Karen" the banner said as it fluttered in the river breeze that came through the opened terrace doors.

"I love it!" I roared. "And I love you! All of you! . . . and I love going to the party!"

Dr. Harris had been right, I thought as my tears spilled freely. Nothing else mattered—I was going to the party.

"Who made the cake?" I cried, dipping my finger in the dark chocolate frosting. "It's fabulous!" The dining room table was laden with all of the items I had requested during my hospital stay: prosciutto, melon, artichokes vinaigrette, Godiva chocolates, fat red plums, translucent green grapes—it was all there. The unorthodox menu for this feast had been assembled with only one organizing principle: indulge Karen.

And that, I soon saw, was to be the prevailing attitude for the day. Indulge Karen. Whatever Karen wants, Karen gets.

The phone would ring. "It's Linda," my mother said, her hand covering the mouthpiece, "do you want to talk?"

"Yes."

"Okay, Linda, she wants to talk."

I would finish my coffee. "Do you want more coffee, honey?" Neill would ask. "I'll make another pot."

I would rub my eyes. "Do you want to rest, Mom?" Adam would ask charitably. Do you want a drink? Do you want to open your get-well cards? Do you want to change your clothes? Do you want to go out on the terrace? Do you want the flowers in your bedroom? Oh. What's that? You want to go to the bathroom? Wonderful! Terrific! She wants to go to the bathroom.

When I could no longer suffer their indulgence, I went quietly to my bedroom, closed the door, and lay down on the bed; I half expected to find they'd installed a call button in the headboard.

Instead, they'd unpacked the brand-new yellow-and-white-flowered linens that were to have been opened in California and made up the bed and room with the style and panache of a Bloomingdale's catalog page. Flowers from my room at Neuro covered every available surface. It was like falling asleep in a garden. Melinda Marks would have loved it.

Neill leaned over me and handed me a glass of water. "I'm sorry to wake you," he said, "but you'd better take the Decadron now. McMurtry was very concerned that you follow the dosage schedule for the next few days."

I sat up and swallowed the pills. "How long did I sleep?" I mumbled. The clock radio was obscured by a bunch of pink and white carnations.

"About three hours. Would you believe your mother is already getting dinner together?" he laughed.

"That's her coping strategy, Neill," I said. "Don't knock it; it works for her."

"I'm not knocking it," he said, licking his lips, "I'm enjoying it." But there were fine spidery lines around his eyes when he looked at me, and his mouth was rigid when he smiled.

"What's *your* coping strategy, my darling?" I said, trying to bring his face into sharper focus. "I sleep, and my mother cooks, and my father reads to the kids. What do you do?"

"I love my wife," he said soberly.

"Then do it," I whispered against his chest. "Do it now. Go lock the bedroom door, and do it."

"I thought you'd never ask," he said, shedding his clothes and diving into bed. "All that talk about coping strategies? It didn't sound like you. It sounded phony," he said as he began to touch my breasts. "Like something from one of Edye's textbooks."

"You're right," I laughed, feeling my body respond in a thousand star bursts, "it ain't my style, that jargon."

"What is your style, lady?" he said, entering me gently, tentatively.

"Not this, buddy, not today," I growled, wrapping my legs around him. "More like this."

"Easy there, tiger," Neill said, slowing the pace. "Remember your doctor's orders—for the first few weeks I'm supposed to do all the work."

"That ain't my style either, Neill."

The homecoming party, which I had by now named the "relief revels," picked up steam after dinner. People who had hesitated to visit me in the hospital came readily to the house. If I were fit company for my children, they reasoned, I must not be such damaged merchandise after all. I was ready for viewing. So the phone rang, and the intercom buzzed, and they arrived—the people who had been too timid for Neuro. Most of them brought offerings of some sort: champagne, flowers, homemade goodies, and trinkets they knew would be well received by Karen "the Gypsy."

I drank the wine, sniffed the flowers, put on the jewelry, and secretly wondered why no one had thought to bring me books—the mainstay of the get-well gift department. Perhaps they weren't so sure about me, after all. The thought was fleeting, but unsettling in the extreme.

"You look fabulous," Jeff said, when I opened the door. "What did they do to your skin? You look like a Clinique ad." He stood awkwardly in the hallway, afraid to touch me, clutching a bottle of cognac.

"You can hug me, dummy," I said, "I won't break."

"Ach, why take a chance?" he said, walking past me into the living room.

Jeff wasn't the only one. Others, too, kept their distance that night, lavishing compliments from afar, cheering me from a distance. But in my rapturous intoxication with life I forgave them their hesitation and uncertainty and sought to convert them with my own exuberance. I danced, I sang, I laughed, and I freely answered questions. The toughest question of all—"What exactly is wrong with you?"—was my meat, the heart of the "brave me" role.

"Well," I told them, holding out my empty wine glass for more Moët et Chandon, "that is a very, very good question. You see, no one seems to want to tell me." Conversation screeched to a halt. They looked from me to Neill to my parents and squirmed. And I *let* them squirm. My own euphoria could not be disturbed; it was too fragile. Better they should squirm than me.

"We'll know in a couple of weeks," Neill finally said. "It's either a brain tumor or something called aqueductal stenosis." He could be straightforward, I thought as I watched my friends and neighbors flinch. He's wounded, but he's not fragile.

That irreverent combination of Neill's stoic directness and my impeccable jubilance worked. Either the Brownsteins had lost all reason, our guests figured, or Karen was going to make it. Most people left smiling, preferring to think the latter.

Sunday's crowd was a much tougher audience. Mike and Dorrie Margolin had driven in from Moorestown to see me, and friends who happened to be radiologists stopped by at the same time. When Billy Di Mauro rang the doorbell, I began to feel like the Gertrude Stein of the neuro crowd.

Just like the friends who'd come the night before, this group also brought affection and concern, but their caring was enhanced for me by their knowledge. No one in this assemblage needed definitions; all of them could say "brain tumor" without missing a beat. None of them wanted to say it: it just slipped out in conversation. Like the information about Dr. Lissal.

"We've worked with him," the radiologists said as they sipped iced coffee on the terrace. "The man's a true demon in the field. No wonder his associates are afraid to utter an opinion. He'd have them all beheaded and then run a CAT scan on the remains!"

"He *is* the acknowledged expert," Billy said graciously. "If it were my brain, I'd be glad he was available for diagnosis."

"You Italians really are charming," Neill chuckled as he raised his glass of wine. "The problem, Billy, is that he is not available for diagnosis. At least not now."

"How long will you have to wait?" Dorrie asked kindly.

"Dorrie," I answered, "you're terrific. Leave it to the one person who's *not* a doctor to zero in on the heart of the matter. The an-

113

swer to your question is: two, maybe three weeks before he gets back to the States and looks at my films."

The medical contingent sighed with exasperation.

"That stinks," Dorrie said coldly. "That just stinks." Mike stood up and paced the living room. "What does Melinda have to say about that?"

"I was hoping you would tell *me*, Mike," I said, crestfallen.

I T WAS THE BEGINNING OF THE END OF THE PARTY. People still brought gifts, and the phone continued to ring incessantly, but it was never the same after that Sunday afternoon. Princess Admirable was fading fast.

By Wednesday afternoon, the mirror confirmed it. The show-stopper complexion began to erupt; the acne that had graciously skipped me during adolescence made a delayed appearance.

"Boo!" I said to the bewildered face in the mirror. "Who invited you? Bring back the old skin." Over the next couple of days, the empty Decadron bottle on my bathroom shelf was replaced by an array of creams and soaps that were as helpless as I was to explain the change in my complexion.

And the changes were more than skin deep. I was having headaches.

"No," I told Mike over long-distance telephone a few days after he'd visited, "they are not like the ones I had before surgery. But they are there, and they do frighten me." My palm was sweaty against the receiver. Neill stood at the foot of the bed looking tired and grim.

"And Mike," I said apologetically, "I know it's not your territory, but I've been having some chest pain, too. On the left side." I was near tears, biting my lip and rubbing my left shoulder.

"No, I am not playing with the shunt," I exclaimed. "What a bizarre thing to suggest. I'm just a little uneasy, that's all. And I'd rather talk to you than to Marks or McMurtry."

Mike kept me on the telephone for nearly an hour, soothing me, reassuring me, and then suggesting that I call Dr. McMurtry.

"What about the chest pain?" I asked before he could hang up.

"Karon," he said to me in a voice so full of patience and authority

115

that I knew I was getting what he normally reserved for the paying patients, "you've been through one hell of an ordeal. It's normal to be fearful. You're vulnerable right now—anybody who had gone through what you have would be. But let me set you straight on something: you are not having a heart attack. First of all, you are too young and too healthy. Second of all, your body has been gone over with a fine-tooth comb. If there were anything wrong with you below the neck, they'd have found it when you were in the hospital. Now, just try to relax. Don't be afraid to use that Valium you were given in the hospital. And call Jim McMurtry; he'll tell you what to do for the headaches. Okay? Karen? Okay."

"I love you, Mike," I said, tears of relief clouding my vision, "I'm so glad I called you. I really do feel better. I think I'll go wash my precious hair!"

"Ah," Mike laughed. "The long-awaited shampoo baptism ceremony. Enjoy," he said, in the voice of my friend.

"He says the headaches could be withdrawal from the Decadron," I said to Neill when I'd hung up.

"Well," Neill said, his face relaxing into the dimpled smile that framed his mustache, "that certainly makes sense. When did you take the last one?"

"Yesterday . . . I think yesterday." I got out of bed and pulled my nightgown over my head. "I'm going to take a shower and wash all this EEG goop out of my hair. Do you realize it's been in there for two weeks? Yech! Want to help?" I winked.

"No," he said, "it sounds like a private pleasure. Besides, it would shake my manhood to watch a grown woman have an orgasm with a bottle of Breck for normal hair."

"Spoilsport," I shouted as I entered the bathroom, "where's your sense of American values? Don't you know that the clean hair fetish is right up there with conspicuous consumption and Medicare?" I stuck my head out of the bathroom.

"You go ahead," he said. "Play with your bubbles. I'll stand by if you need me."

"Your choice," I said, as I closed the opaque shower door. I took a deep breath, adjusted the shower head to full throttle, arranged my body so that my head was clear of the spray, and pulled the knob.

Oh, God, I thought as the warm water sluiced over my skin, life is glorious. No more stranger's hands wiping me with damp washcloths that smell of alcohol. No more contortions at that ugly little sink. I'm home!

I took the cap off the shampoo and let the water pour over my head, but memory washed over me with a velocity far stronger than the water. The shunt, the pneumo, the arteriogram—I relived all of it, as the water splashed off my hair. Massaging my head tenderly at first, I piled up the rich lather so that my fingers made no contact with my scalp. So much hair! What was it Dr. Harris had said when I'd asked him how my new hair would grow in if it were all lost in radiation treatments? There was some word he'd used to describe it, some very unscientific adjective that had made me laugh at the time. What was it?

My fingers touched the small hollows in the back of my skull. The burr holes, I thought, as I carefully traced their dented periphery with my fingers. I'd made a joke of them when Dr. McMurtry was removing the sutures.

"Can I smoke dope," I'd said, "or will I give the world a contact high through the holes in my head?"

"I'm not rightly sure I know," he'd laughed. "We'll have to look that one up."

I rinsed my hair and lathered my head a second time. "Luxuriant!" That's the word! "It will grow back, Karen, but it will never be as luxuriant as it is now," is what Dr. Harris had said. I poured creme rinse over my head and stroked it through the wet hair. Now I could feel the shunt, a tiny tube protruding just slightly from my scalp behind my right ear.

Aw, no, I cried silently, beginning to give way as my soapy hands explored the damaged terrain of my skull. I don't want to lose my hair. I don't want to go back there any more. I want it to be over. Please, dear God, let it be over.

While my tears fell in torrents, I screamed against the rush of the water, "Enough! God, help me! I've had enough!" I sat down on the tile floor of the shower, the water puddling at my feet, and grieved for the death of Princess Admirable.

"Damn it!" I shouted at Neill as I stood dripping all over the bedroom carpet, "Call Dr. McMurtry and find out why the hell I should be having headaches *now*! And why my skin is ravaged! And why I should still be having double vision two weeks after surgery! Call him!"

117

"Is that an order?" Neill asked, his voice as hard as the stone of Neuro's facade.

"No," I said trembling, "but if you won't do it, I will. I'm tired of all this pain." I lay down on the flowered sheets and buried my clean, wet head under a pillow.

An hour later I had blown my hair stylishly dry, put on makeup, dressed, and was seated at the kitchen table while my mother tried to cajole me into eating something.

"Mother," I said with mock exasperation, "you've got to give up this cooking therapy. You're sabotaging all of my plans. I lost seven pounds in the hospital. I had hoped to lose seven more, bleach my hair blond, and trade Palo Alto for Malibu! How am I ever going to make the cover of the next Beach Boys' album if you keep dosing me with Jewish mother-love?"

My mother had the confused gaze of someone who's gone out for popcorn and missed one of the key scenes in a Hitchcock thriller. She sat down opposite me and took my hand in hers.

"Karen," she began softly, "I can't keep up with you, honey. One minute you're flying, and the next minute you're crying." She closed her eyes and massaged her brow. "And the next minute after that, you're making jokes about California. I don't know which is the real you, Karen." There was such sadness, such bewilderment in her face that I got up and kissed her.

"They're all me, Mom," I said tearfully. "Just keep praying the good girl wins in the end."

Dr. McMurtry returned Neill's call. I was back in bed when the phone rang next to me.

"You get it," I said to Neill, "I don't want to hear this. Go talk to him on the extension in the kitchen."

"You're lying right next to the damn telephone," Neill shouted. "Talk to him, for crying out loud!"

"I don't want to talk to him!" I shouted back.

Neill took the phone call in the kitchen. I lay in bed and tried to will the double vision away.

"Well?" I asked, when Neill came back into the bedroom a few moments later. "What did he say?"

"The same thing Mike said. The headaches are probably the result of withdrawing the Decadron. You can take aspirin for them." He forced a smile.

"And my skin?" I asked angrily.

"I didn't mention your skin," he said.

"Why not?"

"Because I don't give a damn about your skin, Karen. I was more concerned with your headaches."

"You were right," I said resentfully. "What else did he have to say?"

"He said we should both relax and enjoy the Bicentennial."

As the tall ships sailed majestically past our apartment terrace, Princess Admirable breathed her last. No longer were the periods of indiscriminate churlishness and pernicious self-pity redeemed by moments of boundless joy and thoughtful gratitude. So what if America was celebrating her biggest birthday party; for me, the party was over. The princess was dead; no costumed reenactment of the Battle of Concord could resurrect her.

Depression so deep it confounded speech held me in its powerful grip and twisted mercilessly. While my family leaned over our terrace railing and hailed the billowing parade of nations, I sat mute in a chair, reviewing the ships with the stony eyes of the damned.

The *Eagle*. The *Forrestal*. The full-rigged *Amerigo Vespucci*. The spectacular *Esmeralda* from Chile. None of them moved me. Music—brassy Sousa marches and triumphant Tchaikowsky—floated out from other terraces where glass-clinking orgies of patriotism were in progress.

"I don't want to go," I'd told Neill without explanation when he'd pleaded with me to go up to Billy's apartment where our friends were celebrating. "Go without me." But he hadn't gone and now as I sat in my chair, silent and cold as the time capsules buried all over America this day, he was lost to me. All of them were lost to me.

"Look! Mommy, look! It's the *Libertad*!" Adam had risen at four o'clock in the morning to see the ships assemble in New York Harbor. He knew them all on sight.

"Isn't it terrific, Mommy? Isn't it terrific?"

I could not answer my own child. I could not bring the words to my lips, so profound was my depression.

"What does it mean, Mom? *'La Libertad'*?"

"It means liberty, honey," my mother said, watching me sorrowfully. "It means freedom, independence." Adam watched me, too, waited for me to come around. It was the greatest extravaganza in the nation's history; surely his mother would soon drop this awful charade and enjoy the celebration. When at last Adam gave up on me, he turned his back defiantly and continued to identify the ships.

"I'm going back inside," I said. The suddenness of my voice made everyone start.

"Me too, Moomie," Todd said as he stretched his arms to be carried. His face, sticky with a red, white, and blueberry Good Humor, beseeched me.

"No," I said tonelessly, and walked through the terrace doors into the empty apartment. "Let me be." No one followed.

I got into bed and pulled the yellow comforter around me, but it offered no warmth. Nothing gave comfort to me on this day. While the ships came about on the river outside my window, I could think only of them, the white coats, just a few miles downriver behind their stone wall. Somewhere in that building my future was hanging in a gray X-ray envelope, untouched, unattended.

"What's taking them so long!" I demanded when my mother came in and sat on the edge of the bed. "I can't wait any longer. It's not fair!" And then the unbidden silence again, rupturing the day like death.

"Karen," my mother said. "Try to be patient just a little while longer. Dr. Lissal will be back in a week. We'll all be more like ourselves when we know where this thing is going." Her speech was punctuated by the explosion of firecrackers. Icy fingers began to creep across my legs, up my back. They closed around my neck and squeezed until I screamed.

"What?" my mother shouted. "Tell me! What's wrong? Is it pain? Tell me!" Frenzy made her eyes wide and girlish.

It wasn't pain—it was something worse. It was the Crazy Lady, the stranger who had stolen into my body and taken possession. For two days I had worked frantically to cast her out. "Leave me alone," I had hissed when she first came. "I'm doing all right. Just leave me alone. I don't want you." The Crazy Lady only snickered. She'd been snickering ever since.

"You will die," the Crazy Lady announced with her first visit. "Your future is murdered." At first I only believed her. Then, I became her—the catatonic embodiment of defeat.

"Help me!" I screamed to my mother, grabbing both her hands. "There's another woman living in my body! Get her out! I hate her! Mother! She's going to kill me! Get her out! Please!" I began to scream, long piercing syllables of terror.

120

Neill ran into the room, shook me, and cradled me in his arms.

"It isn't her, Neill," my mother whispered, wringing her hands. "She says there's someone else in her body. Oh, my God, my God! Help her!"

Neill held me with one arm and with the other he reached for the telephone. I could not stop that desolate wailing.

"Who are you calling?" my mother asked, her own terror splintering my cries.

"Mike Margolin."

"I don't want to hear!" I screamed. "I don't want to hear! I'm afraid. Oh Neill, I'm so afraid. What if she never goes away? What if she stays with me forever? I can't live with her!"

Neill began to speak, his voice the only calm in the center of this storm.

"Michael," he said quickly, "it's Neill. Karen's having hallucinations, I think. She says there's another woman in her body . . . Since . . ." he pulled me away from him and looked into my eyes, "since when, Karen?"

"Yesterday," I said firmly.

"Since yesterday, Michael." Panic was chipping at the edges of Neill's voice. "Yes, yes. Very depressed . . ." he said into the telephone. ". . . I don't know. You better talk to her." He handed me the telephone. It was cold and slippery.

"Karen?" Mike's voice sounded so far away. "Listen to me, listen to me carefully. When is the last time you took the Decadron?" It had been days, but I was too far gone to be able to count them.

"Days," I choked hoarsely. "A few days, I think."

"All right," he said decisively. "Now get this straight, Karen. There is no other woman living in your skin. You are you. What you are experiencing are the withdrawal symptoms from taking a very powerful steroid. Didn't anybody at the hospital warn you that withdrawal from Decadron could produce these mood swings?" My head lurched against my chest. I dropped the phone.

The Crazy Lady had a name after all. Chemical depression—depression brought on by withdrawal from a drug. Not from a brain tumor, not from aqueductal stenosis, not by a rend in my consciousness that had allowed the stranger to sneak in and wreak havoc. Chemical depression—chaining me to fear, starving my courage, freezing my voice. No, no one had warned me. No one had even hinted.

"Enjoy the Bicentennial" had been the last message from Neuro.

WAITING ONCE MORE ON AN ORANGE NAUGAHYDE CHAIR, I was in the basement of Neuro to have my "after" pictures taken. It was hoped that a second CAT scan, to be compared with the one taken before the shunt was installed, would bear witness to the success of my bread-and-butter surgery.

Neill and I sat and leafed through the same dismal old copies of *Sports Illustrated* that I had used as a shield against John Ubeleski's questioning stare three weeks earlier.

I reached for Neill's hand. "I'm glad it's you," I said softly.

"And I'm glad it's *you*," he said, kissing the tip of my nose. "I have to admit it, being married to the Crazy Lady was no fun!" We both laughed, the belly-deep laughter of relief. There had been the threat of a real twister in my brain; instead, it had turned out to be a chemically seeded squall.

"Hey," Neill said, squinting, "I think that's Dr. Harris at the other end of the hall." I stood up and looked down the hall, the same hall in which I'd lain signing release forms for the pneumo-encephalogram and the surgery.

"Hey! You! Dr. Kildare!" I called. "Come on down here and say hello."

Dr. Harris came striding down the hall, his smile wide in greeting.

"Well, how's it going, Karen?" he said, shaking my hand vigorously, but asking the question with no real interest.

His smile was as warm and his manner as personable as ever, but it was clear in the way he shuffled his feet that I was no longer his case. New exotica had claimed his attention since I had left the hospital; learning was proceeding nicely without me.

"How is it *going*?" I repeated, trying to smooth the cutting edge of my voice. "Well, Dr. Harris, to be perfectly candid, there have been a few rough spots." I smiled, disarmingly, I hoped, and moved in for the kill.

"For example, doctor, withdrawing from Decadron? Hmm?" I let the question and the poisonous tone in which I'd asked it dangle in the space between us before I continued. "I find it quite regrettable that you could discharge me from the hospital just in time for me to go stark raving mad in full view of my children!"

"Well," he laughed awkwardly, "you don't think we want to sit around and watch you go crazy here, do you?"

"If that's a joke, Dr. Harris, it isn't very funny," Neill said coldly. "If you couldn't warn Karen of what to expect, you might have at least told me." Dr. Harris looked at the scuff marks on the floor.

"Look," Neill continued, struggling to maintain control of his temper, "we understand that patients are highly suggestible after an ordeal like Karen's. Mike Margolin has made that point repeatedly. I know that if you had told Karen there were ten possible side effects of that drug, no matter how remote the possibilities in her case, she would probably have experienced at least eight of them. She was that vulnerable, I agree. But that doesn't answer for me! That doesn't explain why I had to sit by and wring my hands believing that my wife had the genuine crazies! Why the hell didn't you warn me? It was godawful frightening."

"Yes, I'm sure it was," Dr. Harris said soberly. His eyes could not meet Neill's. "I guess all of the doctors on your case just assumed that somebody else along the way had indicated there could be mood swings as you were coming off the drug. I guess we got our signals crossed if no one told Neill or you." He shrugged unhappily.

"You know, doctor," I said, sitting down again in the orange chair and motioning him to join us, "I like you. I really do. I liked you even when you gave me that charming nonanswer about the blue dress and the pink dress. I thought you had more than medical expertise, I thought you had style: bedside manner, if you'll pardon the cliché." He smiled self-consciously. "And even though what you describe as 'mood swings' felt like catatonic schizophrenia to me, I still like you." I sighed and watched Neill. He knew me well enough to know that this scene was not yet played out.

"But what I don't like, Doctor, what I cannot accept is 'crossed signals.' That's not only a lousy defense, it's a blood-chilling account of what can happen when a patient is at the mercy of a teaching hospital!"

Laboratory errors, misplaced records, fruitless and exhaustive testing—these could occur in any medical establishment; but the catastrophic consequences of "crossed signals"—less than perfect communication among people jointly responsible for a patient—seemed especially ominous in a gigantic medical center, where hordes of overworked and underpaid residents and scores of inexperienced interns had such easy access to patients.

"There's got to be a better way," Dr. Harris agreed without embarrassment. "Maybe it will come to you while you're having the CAT scan." He stood up. "In the meantime, how *are* you doing?" Perhaps he only meant to shift the conversation to a safer subject, but this time I thought his interest was genuine. I still liked him.

"Ah'm doing jus' fine," I drawled, in tribute to his chief, Dr. McMurtry. "And ah'm doin' even better for having said my piece. Thanks for asking." We shook hands again and said good-bye. He was due in surgery and a nurse was calling my name in front of Room B2.

Neill took my arm. "I'll go in with you," he said. He made it sound casual, but I heard the offer as an invitation to dependence. I could handle a CAT scan on my own, thank you. God knows I needed no more opportunities to play the damsel in distress than had already been too amply provided.

"No, you won't" I said, unhooking my arm from his and facing him squarely. "First of all, I have a few things I want to say to that machine privately. I have a feeling that no matter what those pictures show today, Neill, the CAT and I have a long future together. I think we need to get acquainted, the old CAT and I. Besides, you're not fooling me, pal. You know you can't stay in the room once they turn on the juice. What you're after is a little peek at the machine, right? You sneaky old high-technology investment analyst, you. You don't fool me. You just want to see if the name on the scanner is one of your deals or not. Go up and visit with Billy, instead. I'll see you when it's over."

So I went in alone—as I had the first time, but so much more at ease that I looked around the waiting area hoping to play John Ubeleski's brave veteran role to someone else's anxious rookie. There was no one waiting. And no technician in the room. I sat down on the table and looked at the angular equipment.

"Having a slow day?" I said to the beige machine that took up nearly half the room. "Things getting monotonous for you? I know just how you feel, CAT. All this waiting around can really get you down. So do me a favor, will you, scanner? I know you can do it, everyone around here keeps telling me you're the guy with the goods. Deliver, will you? Please? Give me a set of pictures that can set me free."

The machine obliged me. An hour and a half later I stood with Neill in front of an illuminated panel that boasted the most gorgeous set of "before" and "after" pictures a woman could wish. The cloud of fluid that had obscured my brain in the presurgery films had completely vanished!

"Actually," said the radiologist who, along with Neill, had urged me to study the films, "actually you have very small ventricles, as it turns out." It was spoken like a compliment, as though he were praising some other, more pedestrian area of my anatomy, like dainty feet. Or delicate ears.

"Well, then," I said as I drew deep breaths, "there doesn't appear to be any tumor there, does there? All you've pointed out to me is a lot of healthy brain tissue, a small but expensive tube, and adorable ventricles. Is that it?" No one answered. There were three diagnostic radiologists in the room and not one spoke. The light in the panel hummed, Neill coughed, and I waited for someone, anyone, to speak.

"When Dr. Lissal returns he will make the diagnosis," a voice with a slight European accent finally said from behind me.

"Who are you?" I asked, whirling around. A short, squat man in a white jacket answered.

"I work with Dr. Lissal." The words were deliberate, but the tone was ambiguous. Perhaps I had come upon the one brave foot soldier who would speak for the absent general in time of crisis.

"Well, then, you know my case?" I said, leading him.

"Yes. I know it."

"Wonderful! Then you can look at today's scan and tell me there's no brain tumor there, can't you?"

"No. I cannot."

"Why not? For God's sake, why not?"

"Because I am not Dr. Lissal."

———————
———————
———————

Dr. Lissal returned two days later. He studied my films and said just two things: "pinealoma" and "radiation therapy." He may, in fact, have said much, much more, but those words alone

125

constituted the ominous message I received that summer afternoon when Dr. McMurtry called my home. I was alone when the call came.

The diagnosis was not what made me dizzy as I clutched the telephone; far more unsettling to me at the time was the fact that I was hearing these words secondhand. Never in all of my sweat-soaked fantasies of this moment, had I ever imagined that the words might not be spoken by Lissal himself. In all of my dreams, it was he who shook the death rattle.

Three weeks is enough time for an endangered brain to do a lot of thinking; even a feathered Princess Admirable could have figured it out with a minimal amount of research on pinealomas and aqueductal stenosis. The diagnosis was not clear-cut.

"It's ambiguous, isn't it?" I'd said to my friends who were radiologists. No one had said yes and no one had said no. But all of my carefully rehearsed challenges to the diagnosis went down the tubes when I heard Dr. McMurtry's sad drawl.

"Dr. Lissal believes there is a tumor in the pineal gland of your brain and that five thousand rads of cobalt radiation therapy is the proper treatment."

"And you, Dr. McMurtry," I said between deep breaths, "what do you believe?"

"I believe you ought to follow his advice, Karen." I owed Dr. McMurtry my life; it was impossible not to trust him. Were it not for his surgical skill, that cloud of cerebrospinal fluid might still be engulfing my brain even as we spoke. From the beginning I had cast him as the hero in this real-life drama. It was not his fault that in the eleventh hour he had been made to carry the dagger; that was Lissal's doing, and I found it unforgivable.

"I gather Dr. Lissal will be calling me soon," I said with far more confidence than I felt.

"Uh, no," said Dr. McMurtry. "I doubt it. These things usually follow a certain pattern. Dr. Wong's office will be calling you."

"Dr. Wong? Who is Dr. Wong?"

"He is the chairman of Therapeutic Radiology. They have had marvelous—"

"I know," I interrupted him brusquely, "they've had marvelous results with pinealomas. You told me." So now "they," or at least one of them, had a name—Wong. And soon the name would have a face. Only the unfathomable Dr. Lissal remained faceless, voiceless, unknown, and all powerful.

"Thank you for delivering the message," I said when I was able to get past the irony of the words.

"It's not a message I had hoped to bring you, Karen," he said in that long-spun way of his. "But I do think it's best that you go ahead with the radiation now . . . rather than have regrets later." There was a finality in his voice that made me shiver. From this point on he would not be in charge of the file labeled "Karen Osney Brownstein." The future of this case would unfold behind doors of lead. He would not be with me there.

"I'll miss you, Dr. McMurtry," I said. "I don't suppose you could fix it so that I get a machine that buzzes with a Texas accent, could you?"

He laughed appreciatively. "I'll miss you, too," he said. "You're an extraordinary patient, Karen. But I'll stay in touch. And I'll see you before you head out west."

"Yes," I said, "stay in touch."

The certain prospect of radiation triggered a new set of fears and prompted a whole new line of questioning.

To begin with, I was suddenly and uncontrollably in love with my hair. Until now, I realized, I had taken every strand totally for granted. After all, how much thought do you give to the color of your eyes? Or your perfectly ordinary nose? Unless you're an unashamed narcissist, probably not much. My hair was my vanity, but I hadn't known that until I thought about losing it. I had spent all of those years brushing it, combing it, setting it, and forgetting it. No longer.

I stood in the bedroom with the blower in my hand and wept. Me, with my thick, glossy mop of hairdresser's delight, was about to qualify as a circus freak. Neill, whose own hair was thinning prematurely, sat reading *The New Yorker* and trying to ignore me.

"Why should it matter so much?" I asked him, embarrassed by this rush of self-love. "Why can't I just be grateful that I'm still alive? Why must I cry every time I brush it?"

"Because you love your hair," he answered with perfect honesty. "And I love it, too," he said, putting aside the magazine. "But your hair will grow back eventually. They've all told you that. Mine is going for good. Think of me."

When I did think of him I almost always wanted to cry. While I had filled the weeks since surgery trying to balance between Princess Admirable and the Crazy Lady, Neill had held up our world—

the children, our parents, our friends, and the heaviest load of all—me. Day after day he would go to his midtown office, put on the mask of the successful, dynamic financial analyst, call me three times in the course of the day, and come home early to change his business suits for white tennis shorts, brightly colored polo shirts, and sneakers.

"You have to wear those things," I'd told him. "It's summer. It's my favorite season and I'm missing it this year. You must be my summer." A year later he would write to me:

Holding all of us together was a burden, like crossing a desert without water. The unending summer gave us so few succulent leaves to chew on . . . I felt so lonely . . . like a spaceman launched into orbit without the customary electronic communications. . . . My dearest, I stretched my arms beyond their limits to hold you so tightly in the center of that holocaust . . . so that you might see only the sunlight piercing through the eye of the storm. . . .

While Neill succeeded most valiantly in his self-cast role as Atlas, I failed miserably as Karen, the medical investigator. Two days before my scheduled consultation with Dr. Wong, I was still trying to persuade the doctors that the test results were fuzzy, inconclusive; that maybe, just this once, Dr. Lissal might be wrong. Perhaps my questions were too pointed, too threatening to the code of the profession, but nobody was willing to contradict the star. The most anybody would concede was that it was better to be safe than sorry. "Go ahead with the radiation," said Drs. McMurtry, Margolin, and Di Mauro. But they were my friends. How could they possibly see the truth?

As for the great one himself, I had waited in vain for the elusive Dr. Lissal to return half a dozen phone calls in which I'd begged and pleaded to speak with him. "He does not interact with patients," I was finally told by an unidentified voice whose European accent was eerily familiar. The world-famous Dr. Lissal would neither see me nor speak to me. He was more like the Wizard of Oz than even I had imagined.

No, no one messed with the Wiz. Except perhaps . . . I had one shot left. For the straight poop I needed the straight shooter: Melinda Marks.

On the night before I was to meet with Dr. Wong I asked her the single question that had haunted me for weeks: "What if it turns out that there is no tumor in my brain, and I have the radiation therapy anyway?"

"You get your brain fried for nothing," Melinda Marks said.

You want straight talk, you go to a straight talker. For all that her words frightened me, I trusted her candor. Of all of my doctors, friends included, Melinda Marks alone seemed to understand this awful fear—fear of being a patient in a teaching hospital, a research institution.

"Let me tell you something, Karen," she said to me that night. "Radiation therapists love their work."

"I thought most folks in medicine loved their work," I answered.

"That's true," she'd said. "But not like those research guys. I mean they really *love* what they do. If they could get me to lie still long enough, they would cheerfully cook my brain. One more cure for their statistics."

H AND IN HAND WE STOOD IN THE SUBTERRANEAN SPACE where the doors were marked "Radiation Therapy." There are such doors in hospitals all over the world. Beyond them lies the future of medical treatment. They are labeled variously: "Radiation Therapy," "Nuclear Medicine," "Chemotherapy," "Laser Therapy," "Instrumental Medicine."

Millions of us will walk through such doors and have to trust our lives to equipment so sophisticated it may cure us without ever knowing our names. I, who was so daunted by things mechanical that I had difficulty changing a battery in a Star Wars toy, was about to place my life—not in the hands of a skilled surgeon, or a brilliant diagnostician—rather, I was about to lay down before a machine. The thought made my head thunder.

We entered a softly lit, richly paneled waiting room full of stylish contemporary furniture. The receptionist's chair was empty. Neill and I were alone.

Neill ran his palm across the dark paneling and whistled. "I'll be damned," he whispered. "It's real wood. A little different than Neuro in decor, isn't it?" he said, looking around.

"Since when are you so taken with appearances?" I asked, lowering my voice as a gray-haired woman wearing a white uniform sat down behind the desk. "They did all right by me at Neuro, you know. Besides," I added, feeling a shiver along my spine, "this place has the look of an expensive Park Avenue funeral parlor. With an air-conditioning system to match. Remind me to bring a sweater—if I ever come back here," I said, as I buttoned the top buttons of my gauzy blouse.

The gray-haired woman looked up.

"Mrs. Brownstein?" she said in that inane rhetorical lilt receptionists use when they know full well you'd rather vanish forever than identify yourself.

"Yes," I said, approaching the desk. She handed me a ball-point pen and several forms, and told me that I could leave them completed on her desk. Dr. Wong was going to be just a few moments late. I could wait right here. She excused herself.

The forms, mostly having to do with insurance, took no time at all. But Dr. Wong took forever. At last, the same woman reappeared and announced that Dr. Wong would see us now.

"Right through those doors, dear," she said, pointing to two forbidding metal doors that miraculously slid apart with a mechanical hum. There was another set of metal doors thirty feet beyond the first. These, like the others, opened electronically. Dr. Wong was standing behind them.

He greeted us with a pleasant hand-shake and a wide, toothy smile that unnerved me completely. What was he smiling about? Melinda Marks's words—"they love their work"—resounded in my brain as he ushered us into a small examining room and closed the door.

He administered a brief, efficient neurological examination; yet another hand now turned off the lights, held the opthalmoscope to my eyes, and pronounced the shunt a success.

"Nice," said Dr. Wong as he snapped on the lights. "Very nice. Nice and flat, your eyes."

"Yes," I said, hearing my own voice as if from a distance. "Dr. McMurtry has done a marvelous job. We are deeply grateful to him, and to his associates as well." "His associates," I repeated to myself. Why did I sound so stiff? Why couldn't I simply say "Dr. Harris" when that was clearly who I meant? I was coming off like Princess Admirable holding court. What was there about this perfectly cordial man that caused my speech to become so formal in his presence, my manner so coldly reserved?

As he spoke knowledgeably of radiation therapy that afternoon there was the tone of the academic in Dr. Wong's voice, the aura of the lecturer about him. It was as though this were the first day of a new semester and he was the learned professor outlining his favorite course. That, in fact, was the word he used to describe the treatment—"course."

"The course of the treatment," he said, glancing at his notes briefly, "will be five thousand rads of cobalt radiation. During the first weeks of the program the radiation will be to the whole head." He punctuated his words with frequent smiles and continued.

131

"Then, in the later treatments, we will radiate the tumor bed through three ports. Those final treatments will concentrate the radiation in the pineal gland."

As he spoke those words, I knew at once what was causing me to hide behind ceremony and politeness: I was there under false pretenses. I had come expecting a consultation; Dr. Wong thought it was All Systems Go. His had been an enthusiastic and confident preview, but I did not want to take his "course." Fascinating though his "program" might be, I did not care to enroll. Like a student who blunders into the wrong classroom on the first day of school, I needed to raise my hand and ask to be excused. At once. I found it impossible to do either, so I kicked Neill, one of those sharp, unobtrusive kicks that serve married people as code message for "Help! Do something quick! I'm in trouble! Save me!" Neill picked up the signal immediately.

"Now, hold on there a minute, Dr. Wong," he said with an impudence that startled the doctor. "No one has ever been able to tell us definitively that Karen has a brain tumor. I have spoken with doctors in California as well as New York. The radiologists in California at Stanford University Medical Center who know about her case are not nearly so anxious to proceed as you seem to be." Dr. Wong listened and began to smile again. Neill paused, waiting for comment. There was only that smile.

"The California doctors have advised us to make our move and let them take periodic CAT scans. They tell us, Dr. Wong, that if there is a tumor there, it will grow. Eventually it will show up on a scan." Having rendered the closing argument for the defense, Neill sat back in his chair and folded his arms. Dr. Wong eyed each of us briefly before he spoke.

"There *is* a tumor there," he said, with a smile that gave new meaning to the cliché of the inscrutable Oriental. "It is the size of an olive."

He said it with such assurance, such authority, that I knew our case was lost for good.

"The size of an olive?" I repeated. "Green or black, Doctor?"

"Green," said Dr. Wong, still smiling.

I flashed on a martini shaker full of cerebrospinal fluid and followed Dr. Wong to the treatment room. Neill lagged behind us, his head hung low. For all of his efforts, all of his long-distance phone calls to far-away medical centers, he could not save me from what was to come.

Dr. Wong had dismissed the opinions of the California doctors

132

with the magnanimous confidence of the president of Hertz repudiating Avis. Let them try harder, his smile seemed to say. We're still number one.

"You know, Mr. Brownstein," he had said to Neill, "you are perfectly free to make that choice. But you must know that we at Columbia have had more experience with pinealomas than almost all other medical centers in the world. But of course, it is your decision." This had been said with no rancor; it was only the civilized voice of a man who believed in his work and loved doing it.

Beyond one set of lead doors was a large open space that contained elaborate monitoring equipment for each of the treatment rooms beyond it. Pausing before a small control panel, Dr. Wong began an expansive explanation of the timing device, the emergency stop system, and the closed circuit television screen that allowed the technicians to view the patient while the treatment was in progress. Although Neill seemed to take some comfort from the equipment and its purpose, the entire explanation was lost on me. I stood frozen at the nearby doorway of the treatment room.

You've come a long way, baby, I said to myself as I stood on that threshold, but you've still got a long way to go.

It had started out as bread-and-butter surgery, but thanks to "maximum efficiency talent distribution," it was coming up French toast. Neill took my hand as we crossed the final lead threshold.

Here was the largest treatment room I had ever seen. Even the oppressive machine that stood at its center seemed dwarfed by so much space, so much emptiness. The hard, narrow table on which I was made to lie while measurements of my head were carefully taken, seemed to float in a space without edges. I lay rigid on the table in the darkened room as the lighted eye of the machine moved mechanically to a position above my head. Just as I reached for Neill's hand, the machine began its slow motored path to the side of my head and beamed its white light against my cheek. "This part of it," I said with studied nonchalance, pointing to the cameralike lens that was aligned with my head, "is almost like a dental X-ray." I looked up at Neill and forced a weak smile—my way of telling him I was all right. But my hand was icy in his, and my breath was labored as the machine hummed its way to the opposite side of my head and still more measurements were taken.

"It's just that great big thing behind me that makes me a little nervous," I said, hearing the timorous voice of a threatened Princess Admirable. "What's that for, anyway?"

"That is the radiation source," Dr. Wong said as he tilted my chin without looking at me. "We're going to take some simple X-ray films now, Mrs. Brownstein. Please don't move once we've left the room." The machine was directly over my head again. I could see the cross hairs of the lens distincty. I closed my eyes against the blinding white light.

Cold and still as a statue I lay and listened to the sounds of their footsteps moving away from me.

"Is this a treatment?" I called as I heard the door pulled open. It couldn't be. It was too soon. Oh, much too soon. I wasn't ready.

"No, no," said Dr. Wong, "just an X-ray to check your position. Now, please don't move." And the door closed with a sound so final I shall remember it all of my life. The lights came on in the room, there was a brief, buzzing noise, and then it was all over. The door opened, the room lights switched off again, and there were living, breathing people at my side.

"We'll wait to check the films," Dr. Wong said as he looked carefully at the position of my head.

While we waited, Dr. Wong and Neill carried on a technical dialogue that was in all ways over my head. While Neill seemed totally at ease with the scientific explanations being given, I screened out those words that had no meaning for me and focused on those that did.

The word that I found most intriguing in their conversation was "block." A special block would be constructed for me. No kindergarten model this—rather, a lead piece that would be made to fit the machine in such a way that only that portion of my head meant to be radiated would actually get zapped. All of this measuring and the tedious sessions of measurement that followed were an effort to keep those invisible wave forms in their place. Without a block, the radiation was a deadly derailed train, a runaway wreaking havoc in my brain. Alignment, perfect alignment between my head and that machine was the ticket to a safe journey. Let them measure all they want, I thought. Let them calibrate their little hearts out.

Another word that captured my imagination was "setup." Once my head had been properly aligned with the machine they would take an X-ray of the "setup," a further precaution I found extremely reassuring. In fact, there was nothing in what they said that alarmed me; all of it was a variation on the theme of precaution. I began to relax as Dr. Wong went off to examine the X-ray just taken.

My legs were stiff with tension when I moved them and my hands wet with perspiration when I let go of the table's edges. I was cold and my back ached from having lain so long on the hard table, but my mind—my mind felt surprisingly at ease. My breathing had become even again, and my voice was normal as I teased the attractive technician, a diminutive, efficient young woman named Pat.

"What's a nice girl like you doing in a place like this?" I said, when she allowed me to sit up for a moment. With her soft brown eyes and her warm, good-humored manner she seemed grossly misplaced in this grim chamber. Almost as misplaced as I. Although she, at least, had the good sense to wear a warm sweater to work in the middle of summer.

"This room is like a deep-freeze," I said to her as I rubbed my hands together. "How do you you stand it?"

"It has to be that way," she said, "to counteract the heat given off by the equipment." "Equipment." Such a lovely, benign word for such a monstrous machine.

"Will you be here throughout the . . . course?" The course was to last six weeks, with a four-day time-out after the third week. Every weekday I would be taking the elevator marked "Radiation Therapy," following the signs, and passing through the lead doors to this room.

"Yes," she said rather cheerfully, "I'll be here." I thought for a moment of what it must mean to come here by choice, to spend one's days willingly in this underground space. I admired Pat; I was pleased that she would be with me.

"They're ready to do a test now," Pat said when Dr. Wong approached. I lay back down on the table, but this time I didn't need to grip its edges.

The test, Dr. Wong explained, would be a simulation of an actual treatment. I would need to lie still for more than three minutes, the length of a treatment. Did I think I could do that? Yes, of course.

"Fine," he said as he made the final adjustment of my head and the machine that loomed above it. "Please do not move at all now, Mrs. Brownstein. Do not move, please, until you hear the door open. We will all be watching you on the monitor." Neill leaned down and kissed my head and they all stepped out, the lights coming on as the door closed with that awesome, solid thud.

For twenty seconds the room filled with a hush so perfect it was palpable, textured. The only sound audible was my own breath-

135

ing. Two staccato clicks ruptured the silence. The clicks were immediately followed by a low, steady hiss that filled the chamber.

I had never felt more alone, more isolated than in those 3.2 minutes. This is only a test, I reminded myself. There is no radiation being delivered. This is a simulation, not the real thing. There is nothing to be afraid of. They are watching you on the monitor. You're doing just fine. Think about your breathing. Count your exhalations. Pretend this is a contest: if you don't move, if you manage to fidget not at all, there will be a reward waiting for you. A prize to honor your achievement. Think of the prize. That's it. This is a test. You are an achiever. Lie still and achieve. This is only a qualifying round, Karen. But pass this, baby, and in three days you'll be ready for the main event. Thatta girl, Karen. Keep breathing.

There were two metallic clicks and the hiss ceased. It was over. The test was over.

"Excellent," said Dr. Wong as he entered the room. "Truly excellent, Mrs. Brownstein. You did not even blink. You will be a fine patient."

So, I had pleased him. I had willed myself into a stillness that was, God help me, admirable. I had swallowed my outrage, gagged on my fear, and come up a winner. I'd qualified for his course. Today was Friday. On Monday, I would be enrolled.

_____

_____

_____

Having learned the lesson of side effects the hard way with the Decadron, I was relentless in pressing Dr. Wong about the side effects of radiation therapy.

"Very few," he said in reply. "Some nausea, perhaps some vomiting. But that is not true of every case."

"What is true of every case?" I asked him.

"Hair loss," he said without smiling. "You will positively lose your hair. It happens in every case. You will not notice it in the beginning of treatment, but it will happen before the course is over. You must not think that it will not happen to you. It will." He had paused, waiting for me to assimilate his words. When he continued, his smile had returned. "But your hair will come back. That is also true in every case."

"When? When will it come back, doctor?"

"Approximately one year. These are transient side effects."

One year did not seem all that transient to me, but I let that pass.

"When my hair comes back, will it be . . . well, what I mean is, will it be the same as the hair I have now?" Or would it not be worth the wait? Would wigs become a permanent part of my life, a shaggy, ever-present prosthesis?

"You have very beautiful hair, Mrs. Brownstein," Dr. Wong said. "When the new hair replaces it, it will not be so . . . luxuriant."

I laughed out loud. "That's in a book, isn't it?" I said.

"I beg your pardon?"

"That word—'luxuriant.' It's in a textbook somewhere, isn't it?"

"I don't recall," he said, clearly confused by all of this attention to semantics.

"Never mind," I said. "So much for the side effects. Now tell me about the risks."

"The risks?"

"You know, Dr. Wong. The dangers. The risks. The bad stuff."

"The risks are minimal," he said quickly. "I am sure Dr. McMurtry has told you: we have a great deal of experience with this type of brain tumor and our results have been—"

"Marvelous?" I said. "Your results have been marvelous."

"Yes. Exactly."

"Fine," I had said, extending my hand in farewell. "I'll be back on Monday. I shall expect your results to be marvelous."

RADIATION IS A PERVERSE FORM OF THERAPY: with almost all other types of medical treatment, the patient waits hopefully to feel better. In radiation therapy, you keep waiting to feel worse. Everyone associated with my "course" held out the same intractable promise: you won't get better until you get worse. You won't even notice the vile side effects of the cobalt beamed at your brain in the early days of your treatment; you will suffer them increasingly over time.

For radiation, I was told repeatedly, is cumulative. It does not work its dark magic all at once. No—it takes time and patience.

I was short on both. Never in my life had I been easily patient. To be long-suffering or, at the least, dispassionate, is not my idea of a life well lived. Far better to err through action than to harbor regrets of opportunities lost. It was Dad's old advice: you can't hit 'em if you don't swing at 'em. In self-help books, I am known as a risk-taker.

There were exceptions, of course. Times when I stuck my fist in my mouth and held on. Times when things were worth waiting for: the evolution of a shimmering love affair; the growth of a full-term pregnancy; the creation of a short story. For these I had time and infinite patience. Why not? These offered results—wholesome, satisfying results.

But radiation therapy? Patience for radiation therapy? It seemed to me impossible to be forbearant in an atmosphere that was touted as curative but felt so destructive.

When I entered the patients' waiting room inside the first set of lead doors the next Monday morning, the scene I encountered was surreal: the patients sat, silent and empty-eyed. Hiding behind magazines. Supporting their steroid-bloated faces with trembling hands. Slumped in stuporous sleep. The "congregation of the damned."

In every way I felt myself to be an imposter here. In search of the dance company for *Singin' in the Rain,* I had mistakenly bungled my way onto the set of Fellini's *Satyricon.* Now, as during that first walk through the halls of Neuro, I had the overwhelming sense of not belonging here. Of being apart. As far as I was concerned, I had nothing in common with the desolate souls that shared the ubiquitous orange Naugahyde seats with me. *They* were sick. *I* was healthy.

What the hell was I doing here, anyway? Not only had it been nearly four weeks since my surgery; I had never even considered myself *sick.* All of those words descriptive of illness and infirmity seemed grossly inappropriate when applied to my case. Through all of this, I had never been infected, impaired, or diseased. What I had been was *thwarted.*

I was a woman full of conceptions and new beginnings who now found herself in a place where things ended. "Terminal," I whispered to Neill. "They all look so terminal."

As if to prove me wrong, the inner mechanical doors slid apart and out trotted a tall, shamelessly fit man in his middle forties. Fascinated, I watched him as he jogged toward the elevator.

"I'll be right back," I said to Neill. "I need to talk to that man." I chased him down the hall, afraid that the elevator might arrive and swallow him up before I could reach him. My heart raced— not from the running—but from the fear that I might lose him. He had to be someone extraordinary. Why else would he be running here? Either he was escaping whatever hideous enterprise went on behind the final door or, unlike the others I had glimpsed, he was surviving it intact. Whichever was the truth, I needed to hear him speak it.

"Who are you?" I asked him breathlessly, oblivious to the impertinence of the question.

"My name is Frank," he said pleasantly, as though he were somehow not surprised to be accosted while waiting for a hospital elevator.

"No, no, I don't mean that," I said. "Are you a patient?"

"Oh," he said, befuddled. "Yes. Yes, I am a patient." The elevator doors opened. I grabbed his sleeve.

"Please," I said, "please don't go yet. I have to ask you something." He let the elevator doors close without entering.

"Thank you," I said, regaining my composure. "Could we talk, please?" There was still so much desperation in my voice that the man looked slightly alarmed. But he stood still and let me go on.

"I'm a new patient," I said softly, as if this were explanation enough for my inexplicable assault.

"Oh," he said smiling with recognition, "I'm an old patient. Tomorrow is my last treatment." Even his broad grin could not contain the joy with which he made that statement.

"Ah," I said, returning his gladness with my own, "so you are both. Both an escapee and a survivor."

"That's right," he said, very pleased. "You've said it so well."

"That's because I'm a writer," I told him for no reason except that this had suddenly become one of the most intimate conversations I'd ever had. "Are you a runner, Frank?"

"Nope," he said sheepishly. "But I'm thinking about taking it up soon. I'm thinking about taking up a lot of new things now that all of this will be behind me."

"You only jog in the halls of radiation therapy?" I laughed.

"So far," he said. "But you gotta start somewhere, I figure." He was like me, this stranger named Frank—a man of new beginnings.. I would be like him—only temporarily thwarted.

"I'm glad to have known you," I said, my voice thick with unspoken feelings. He smiled, and gently touched his hand to mine, like a runner passing the baton. We were teammates, he and I, running in a mysterious relay race. Across the finish line was the beginning.

Three point two minutes, the average time of a treatment. That is all the time it takes. But what a powerful leeching of the soul may be accomplished in 3.2 minutes.

It was not the way the machine looked that scared me when I entered the treatment room that first morning; I never actually focused on the apparatus in the first days of treatment. The lights were always out when I entered the room, and I would pause on the way to the cold narrow table only long enough to hang my lucky jewelry from the metal coatrack, the solitary reminder of a world outside these walls. Apart from the coatrack, the room was barren of all human reference.

I lay on the meager slab of a table in the darkened room and closed my eyes against the slowly approaching light of the machine's eye. So how could I be frightened by what I saw during a treatment? I managed to arrange things so that I saw nothing.

What I couldn't manage to avoid was hearing, and it was this—what I heard during a treatment—that made my heart pound and my blood run cold. It was the silence; a terrible absence of sound that made me quake as I lay on the table.

The impenetrable door would close with the sound of death—"K-chunk!" The hammer that pounds the last nail into the coffin makes a noise that final. Then silence. Until . . . "Click . . . sssssssss," for 3.2 minutes. Until the final "click." That was it. The same awful pattern today as the day before. Silence. "K-chunk . . . click . . . sssss . . . click." Silence. Until the door was opened from the other side, I could not move.

When the door opened it let in the sound of human voices: Pat's light soprano, Neill's mellow bass, Dr. Wong's cordial baritone. The voices from the outside. I felt I could not safely open my eyes until I heard them speak each day.

"You did quite well, Mrs. Brownstein," Dr. Wong said on that first morning. "No different than during the simulation."

Maybe no different to you, buddy, I thought. But to me, this morning's experience had seemed light years away from the pretend game that had preceded it. This morning had been the real thing. It wasn't whipped cream that was coming out of that big baby looming behind me. It was

RADIATION.

I had been locked into this empty room with the real McCoy. Don't kid yourself or me, doctor. I don't care what it looked like on the monitor you were watching out there. You may have been viewing what looked to you like "The Guiding Light" out there on your mini-screen; but in here, it was strictly *Son of Godzilla*.

"There ought to be music," I said while Pat insisted that I lie still as she painted small dots and lines on my face and neck with a deep purple dye to mark the field of my treatment. Another precaution, this one requiring that I modify my hairstyle to cover the dye marks or risk being mistaken for one of New York's expanding population of cult members. Dr. Wong supervised this bizarre face painting with meticulous care.

"I beg your pardon?" Dr. Wong said absently.

141

"Music," I repeated as I felt the cold wetness of the dye on my skin. "Music during the treatment. Something to drown out the sound of the machine."

"Oh, that's not necessary," he said matter-of-factly. "This is not a noisy machine."

Not from where you're standing, pal, it isn't a noisy machine. But just *you* try stretching out on this rack you call a table one day, and let me close that door on you. Then we'll see who thinks music for this room is a good idea and who doesn't!

But I said this only to myself. And at the same time I resolved to solve the problem the same way—by myself.

The next day when the door closed on me and the machine hissed itself into being, a full orchestra struck up the overture to *Fiddler on the Roof*. By the time the door opened, Zero Mostel was just getting into a full-throated rendition of "Sunrise, Sunset."

After all, I figured, if I could lie in Neuro and let my imagination make my own music, I could lie in Radiation Therapy and repeat the trick. Why else had I been collecting and storing song lyrics all of my life? If you can't go to the memory bank and draw on your principal in a crisis such as this, what good is a retentive mind, anyway?

So every day as Neill drove along the river, I selected my music. I began my day by programming for my rapt audience of one.

For a few days, my programming was flawless. Like a good disc jockey, I knew my music and I knew my audience. If my between-song patter wasn't exactly up to network radio standards, at least I was commercial-free. The one thing station WKOB on your stay-sane dial would not tolerate was interruption. I was in the business of furnishing wall-to-wall sound. And like the best of the record spinners from coast to coast, I was always mindful of timing. I needed to fill 3.2 minutes; to come up short was the mark of the amateur. The pros call such programming gaps "dead air."

On the fourth day the music in my head ran out before the treatment was over. Dead air. My body shook so violently in the remaining seconds of silence that it was visible to those watching on the monitor outside. They hit the emergency stop button on the control panel and came flying through the door.

"What happened?" Pat asked frantically. "What's wrong?"

"Nothing," I lied. But I knew that tomorrow I would be changing my format—no more single melodies. From now on, I would use long-playing records: *The Best of the Beatles. Bob Dylan's Greatest Hits. Ella Sings the Blues.* Never again would I risk having to contend with dead air. Radio stations are notorious for overnight changes in format; besides, as the late-night disc jockeys say—"Baby, whatever gets you through the night."

―――――――――
―――――――――
―――――――――

But in a deeper part of my besieged brain I knew that I was *not* getting through the night. I realized that the musical strategy and the refusal to make contact with other patients in the ante-room were related behaviors. Not looking at the machine was a part of it, too. All of it—every bit of the behavior I displayed from the moment I walked through the first set of lead doors until the moment I walked out into the sunlight of Broadway again—was contrived to keep me armed against the perilous reality of what was happening to me. There was more than one kind of "block" operating in my radiation therapy. The block made of lead belonged to *them*; they had confidence in it. The mental block was mine; only I knew how fragile it was.

The dead air incident proved it to me: I needed help. Not the kind of help Neill was giving me by having my treatments scheduled first thing in the morning so that he could accompany me to the inner sanctum before driving to his midtown office. That kind of support seemed universal in radiation therapy: no patients arrived alone during the weeks of my course. Even the in-hospital patients came through the doors with an attendant at their sides or, in most of the cases, behind their wheelchairs.

Initially I had bravely pooh-poohed this loving baby-sitting service of Neill's. I had begun the treatments fully recovered from surgery and I not only talked a good game of "healthy," I felt it as well. Why should Neill have to be inconvenienced daily when the hospital was just ten minutes away? Surely I could drive myself.

"Not a chance," said my husband, "do you have any idea of what your liability would be if you got into an accident and the court knew you were in the process of radiation therapy?"

So much for driving myself to treatments. But it was more than this pragmatic advice that made Neill's morning presence essential to me. With him at my side and my eyes closed, I could pretend that I was anywhere but where I was. I had someone to talk to in the waiting room. Someone to bolster the pretense that I was merely being *thwarted* here.

But I knew better. Even though Neill would hold my hand until

143

the last possible moment, and kiss my head before Pat immobilized it by securing it to the table with surgical tape, I knew better. When the lead door closed, he wasn't there. No one was there— Just me and the machine. The machine knew exactly how to fill the time. I didn't. The machine understood its role perfectly. I was lost in mine. I needed help. Fast.

HOW WOULD YOU LIKE TO GO SHOPPING WITH ME?" I said to Edye when I rang her doorbell on Saturday morning.

"What do you need?" she said, ushering me into her apartment. "Maybe I have it in my refrigerator."

"I doubt it," I said, pouring myself a cup of coffee and sitting down at her dining room table. "What I'm in the market for is not likely to be hiding between the eggs and the milk."

"What's that?" she said.

"Edye, I need two things. A shrink and a wig."

"Oh, my dear," Edye said with a sigh, "you were right. Those are not items I normally keep in stock. How can I help you?"

"You just did," I said. Simply by accepting the fact that I needed her help, and still more simply by offering it without reservation, she had made my peculiar needs seem acceptable.

"Let's start with the wigs," I said. "Let's take a day next week and research the oft-asked-but-never-answered question, Is it true blonds have more fun?" Edye ran her fingers thoughtfully through her own dark brown hair and laughed nervously.

"You make it sound like fun," she said hesitantly. "And, who knows? The answer may be a resounding 'yes, indeed,' but . . ." she swallowed hard, "how are Adam and Todd going to feel about a blond mother?"

"Edye, my darling, intuitive friend, sometimes you are so sensitive it frightens me. That is the very question that prompted the other item on my shopping list—a psychiatrist who can help me deal with the prospect of being not only a bald mother, but a bald woman. If I left it up to Neill, he would gallantly tell me that bald is beautiful! Fortunately, I am more realistic. If I were six feet tall, weighed a hundred and ten pounds, and had cheekbones that wouldn't quit, I might consider high-fashion modeling and forget the wigs entirely. But I am not Verushka—I need wigs. And I need professional advice on how to live for a year as a bald female."

"A year?" Edye said hollowly.

"Yup. That's what the man said."

I was going shopping for a psychiatrist with all of the desperation of a hostess who finds herself out of toilet paper ten minutes before the dinner guests are to arrive. Most people I knew who had shrink-shopped had taken a leisurely stroll through the aisles. They'd had enough time to make careful selections. If the Jungians didn't look especially fresh, or the Freudians were not in season, other people had the luxury of turning their carts full of anxieties and walking down yet another aisle. I had no such luxury; I was your true panic shopper.

"How about my friend Mel at City College? He's sensitive and . . ."

"No," I told Edye, who through her work was well connected with a host of clinical psychologists, "it has to be a *psychiatrist*. Not a psychologist or a social worker. It has to be someone with an M.D. Someone who's been through medical school. Someone with at least a nodding acquaintance with the medical specifics of my case."

"Specifics." I liked that word, and I found myself using it, or variations of it, quite a lot in the next few days while I was in the market for professional counseling. This emphasis on the "specifics" of my case was comforting to me; it set me apart from all of the others who sought private solutions from professional strangers. Or at least I told myself that.

At a time when it seemed to me that almost every one I knew had an analyst, I wanted to make very clear that I was not just one more trendy, self-indulgent young New Yorker, shelling out fifty bucks an hour on the East Side every Wednesday afternoon. There were better things to be encountered on the East Side, I'd always thought: art galleries, first-run foreign movie theaters, and outrageous hot fudge sundaes at Serendipity.

Furthermore, with only one notable exception, no one I knew seemed very much improved by his psychiatric treatment. And it wasn't just the Wednesday afternoon ladies who seemed to be spinning their neurotic wheels, either. For them, a session on the couch was merely a rest stop between their Cuisinart cooking class at Bloomingdale's and their pedicure appointments at Elizabeth

Arden. There were also the people who were seeing doctors four or five times a week and at the same time complaining that their doctors didn't give them enough time. They too seemed to be making little progress in achieving their announced ends.

Maybe that was it. Maybe their *announced* reasons for seeking psychiatric help were not their *real* reasons. Maybe the friend who kept complaining about "free-floating anxiety" (a phrase that invariably made me picture the Goodyear blimp) was really a secret child molester. Perhaps the people who talked long and loud at cocktail parties about such innocent concerns as identity crises and guilt trips were, in fact, latent necrophiles. Who could really say for sure?

But I, with my open and shut case of "specifics," was different. Why, it would take me ten minutes on the telephone just to spit out my specifics to whatever psychiatrist was on the receiving end of my call. And I called only those doctors about whom I'd been previously assured. Everyone I phoned had at least a limited knowledge of what my "problem" was about.

"You're sure?" I'd say to the person who had made the referral. "You're sure I won't call up and have someone say 'Gee, I'd love to help you, honey, but I don't know a pinealoma from a timpani. Try the guy down the block.' "

"I'm sure," they'd say. "He's worked with Elizabeth Kubler Ross."

"Elizabeth Kubler Ross!" I'd holler. "For God's sakes, that's about death and dying!"

Two referrals turned out to be washouts because the doctors at issue were on vacation. A third bombed because the doctor was about to go on vacation. Damn, I thought, my timing stinks. If only I had been consulted about the season of my trauma, I might have been spared the frustration of trying to locate a top-notch shrink in New York City in the summertime. The first string was sailing off Martha's Vineyard and the second team was clamming on Cape Cod at Wellfleet.

These sorry conditions might have been acceptable to someone with an everyday "I hate my mother-I hate sex-I hate myself" syndrome—those poor folks could afford to wait until September. They might whine a lot while they waited, but they could survive. I wasn't so sure about me.

I tried groups; I combed the yellow pages of the Manhattan Directory and located terrific groups for:

        . . . Abused Children
      . . . Child Abusers
        . . . Coronary Patients
        . . . Disaster Victims
        . . . Mastectomy Patients
        . . . Paraplegics
        . . . Rape Victims
        . . . Widows and Widowers

But for me, there was nothing—no Head Club, no Pinealoma Foundation, no Brotherhood of the Brain. Somewhere out there, I kept telling myself, was a person who could help me. Someone who, when familiar with my "specifics," could help me to make it through those 3.2 minutes every day and all of the nights in between. So I continued to search for a psychiatrist.

I thought I had found someone special when I found Dr. Byron. He had been referred to me by none other than Melinda Marks. There were several things that recommended Dr. Byron even before I met him. First, he was a psychiatrist, a medical doctor as well as an analyst. Secondly, I liked the way he *sounded* on the telephone. Not only was his speech slow and sympathetic, he seemed knowledgeable and forthright. Unlike others I had called, he did not seem either condescending or intimidated by a patient who tossed around terms like "ventricular study" or "hydrocephalus" with adandon. In all fairness to those doctors I rejected, I doubt that their phones usually ring off the wall with calls that begin: "I have just had brain surgery, and in six weeks I am moving to California where I will be bald when I meet my new neighbors. Oh, yes, and I must have an afternoon appointment because I spend my mornings having my brain toasted." You really can't blame those doctors for not trying.

But Dr. Byron tried. He let me do the whole ten minutes—the wigs, the kids, the baldness—everything. And then he said a very human, very unpsychiatric word: he said "Wow!" That's what sold me—that "wow!" What also sold me was the fact that he was on the staff of Psychiatric Institute; if nothing else, that at least gave him a neighborly charm.

"I must tell you, Mrs. Brownstein," he said to me in the very first phone call, "that I will not be available to you after mid-August. As much as I would like to be of help to you, I really think you ought to see someone who will available to you for the entire course of your radiation."

148

Son of a gun! He knew about *courses*!

"No chance, Dr. Byron," I said. "You are definitely my guy!"

With the shrink question seemingly answered, I felt free to pursue the wig dilemma. Edye agreed to accompany me to a wholesale wig manufacturer on the West Side of Manhattan.

"Let's make a day of it," I said as we drove into midtown the next Saturday. "I feel great. I managed to get through the entire week of treatments without freaking. And even if that's just beginner's luck, I've got Dr. Byron on deck for Monday afternoon."

"You're on!" Edye said happily. "We'll go get the wigs, hit the first floor of Lord and Taylor, and then what?"

"Trader Vic's!" I answered immediately. "Trader Vic's at the Plaza. A woman with an exotic tumor should definitely have a drink at Trader Vic's!"

The wig trip would have been a lot more fun if the manager of the shop hadn't cried so much and so loudly.

I had hoped to avoid telling her exactly *why* I needed a year's supply of wigs, but from the moment it was clear to her that I wanted several different styles, she became very suspicious.

"What for?" she asked. "Ya got gorgeous hair. Whadda ya wanna cover it all up for? One wig, maybe, I could see it. For after swimming, maybe. But six? Nobody with such hair needs six wigs, sweetheart. Whatsa matter with you?"

I made a big mistake: I told her.

"Oh my God!" she screamed in pure Brooklynese. "Oh my God! . . . Ya got kids?"

"Two," I said, trying to picture my face beneath eighteen inches of jet-black Dynel marked "Cher."

"I don't understand," she whined, handing me another wig, "I don't understand *at all*. You're so young . . . and with kids yet! Oh my God."

"I'm going to be just fine," I said to stop her whimpering. "Could I try on that short-hair one over there? The one with the shaggy bangs?"

"You'll never get it on," she was momentarily distracted. "It'll never fit over all your hair." It was impossible for her to accept that I would, in fact, be wearing all these wigs on my bare scalp.

"Let me try it anyway, please." I said sweetly. "And if you could bring out a few that are just a shade darker I'd appreciate it. These are a little light for me. Hmm?"

149

"Right away," she said, fleeing into the stockroom where she could give full vent to her horror.

"She thinks I'm going to die," I whispered to Edye from beneath a tightly curled number called "Gypsy." "How do I tell her I'm not going to die?"

"You can't tell her, my dear." Edye said. "She'll never believe you. What you have to do is show up here a year from now, sporting your own hair and absolutely oozing good health."

"Edye," I said, "from your mouth to God's ears."

Lord & Taylor was a lot more fun. I bought three huge scarves that were displayed as turbans on mannequins in the hat department. And I took a close look at exactly the way the scarves had been wrapped around the dummys' heads.

"Susan," I said silently, "wherever you are . . . forgive me." Properly wrapped, these scarves would not only hide my baldness, they would also cover the dots of purple dye that peppered my hairline and the back of my neck.

Trader Vic's is a first-rate place to get sloshed. In fact, many of its most loyal patrons are perfectly willing to forgo the marvelous dinner menu, the always crunchy and occasionally profound fortune cookies, and just concentrate on the exotic booze. They toss off the paper umbrellas, the sweet-smelling gardenias, and the candy swizzle sticks the moment the zombies hit the table. Not for nothing are the rest rooms at Trader Vic's well supplied with plenty of antacids and sympathetic attendants.

"You know," I said to Edye as we entered the elegant lobby of the Plaza, "this hotel is my favorite part of New York. In fact, for me, I think the Plaza *is* New York. I'm going to miss it something terrible."

"Relax," she said as we strolled past the Edwardian Room. "I've already booked us a table in the Palm Court for New Year's Eve, my dear."

"You're kidding! You made a New Year's Eve reservation in July?" Edye winked mysteriously and took my arm. We walked down the carpeted stairs behind the Oak Room. At the bottom of the stairs is the tiki-strewn path that leads to the best banana daiquiri this side of the South Pacific.

"We have come to the right place," I said. "The perfect place, in fact. Name one other restaurant in New York that's as appropriate to what we're celebrating."

"What exactly are we celebrating?" Edye asked as she sipped her piña colada.

"Exotica," I said. "We are celebrating exotica. Not only do I have a tumor with an exotic name," I said as I signaled the waiter for another round, "but I'll bet you didn't know that the pineal gland is one of the most romantic parts of the brain."

"Really?" she said with exaggerated fascination as she chewed on a fortune cookie. "Whoever told you that? Your lady neurologist, I bet."

"Nope. Mike Margolin. He was an undergraduate philosophy major. Did you know that Descartes thought the pineal gland was the place where body and soul came together? Isn't that extraordinary? The whole subject of the pineal gland is shrouded in mystery."

"Leave it to you, my dear, to choose a romantic brain tumor. I think we ought to have a toast to Descartes."

As I attempted to raise my frothy glass, I fell sound asleep.

"Karen!" Edye whispered. "What's wrong? Is it the drinks?" I struggled to open my eyes and failed.

"Uh-uh," I mumbled as I lay down in the booth and curled my legs under me, "just shleepy . . . thas all . . . ."

I woke up moments later, finished my drink, and explained to Edye something I had nearly forgotten. One of the lesser side effects of radiation therapy is sudden and uncontrollable fatigue. That, I now realized, is what I had been seeing in all of those slumped patients in the waiting room.

"I have to hand it to you, my dear," Edye said as she finished off her own drink, "you do have class. Who else would have the foresight and élan to pass out in a place where that is totally acceptable behavior?"

"You're right," I said, taking out my fortune. "I am some smart cookie!"

EVEN SMART COOKIES CRUMBLE. They may be more inventive about where they hide their crumbs, but they crumble just the same.

I went to Dr. Byron's office alone, a small triumph of independence. Too bad the glory was undercut by the fact that I took a cab. My abrupt, unexpected nap at Trader Vic's had made me wary of situations where sudden sleep might prove hazardous, or at least inconvenient. I rationalized the $7.00 cab fare by imagining myself falling asleep on the Madison Avenue bus. I could end up riding the bus all the way to the end of the line without realizing my snoozy mistake. Better to take a cab and arrive on time.

I found Dr. Byron's address to be a dingy brownstone in the East 60s. A rickety elevator, walls peeling paint that had once been maroon, carried me to the second floor. I pushed open the elevator door and found myself in an anteroom so small that I instantly knew Dr. Byron didn't treat claustrophobics. Anyone with even a mild case of that particular disorder would have taken one look at this tiny, airless space and bolted for the firestairs.

I had come with cartoon expectations of what a psychiatrist's office should look like: potted palms, indirect lighting, and neat stacks of *The Atlantic Monthly* on a gleaming coffee table. A quiet dignified room, suitable for meditation. Instead, I encountered furnishings that looked like rejects from Goodwill and silence broken by two huge bluebottle flies that buzzed the room like deranged kamikaze pilots.

Nice going, toots, I said to myself. In a neighborhood where all you have to do is stand on the corner and yell "Shrink!" and ten thousand rosewood doors will open, you manage to come up with Dr. Tacky. Wait until your friend Linda hears about *this*.

By the time Dr. Byron opened the door, I expected to see Lucy holding up a sign that said:

And I was sure his opening remarks would be something like: "Around here we don't go in for frills; around here we mostly save psyches."

I was wrong on both counts. Dr. Byron did not look a bit like Lucy; in fact he looked a lot like Yale, class of '55, and his opening remarks were in no way defensive.

"Mrs. Brownstein," he said, "you're early."

While I ticked off a condensed account of my medical history prior to this year, Dr. Byron bent his head over a clipboard and took copious notes. I had given the same accounting so many times, I could do it automatically. As I reeled off the dates of operations and hospitalizations, my mind was free to take in the man and the setting.

The anteroom had been a spurious ruse; *this* room actually had potted plants and soft lighting. It even had the obligatory couch on which I now sat with my knees curled under me. Dr. Byron, sandy-haired and boyish, sat across from me in a black leather wing chair. His eyes were hidden by the gold wire-rimmed glasses that reflected light from the floor lamp beside him.

"Is that all?" he asked as he shook the writer's cramp from his left hand. "Does that bring you up to the present?"

I thought for a moment. I had mentioned my pregnancies, the surgery Dr. Mount had performed on Todd, the emergency abdominal surgery. Had I left something out? Was there more?

"Yes," I said. "That's it. All that's left is my brain tumor." I knew at once I shouldn't have said that; at least not in that glib Princess Admirable tone. I had promised myself that I would not pretty up the picture for Dr. Byron; that I would not hide my pain behind the "smart-assed broad" mask. I did not want to be smart and funny here; I wanted to be honest. Already I was here under false pretenses—on the telephone I had said I wanted to discuss the matter of wigs and small boys. In truth, I wanted to explore and hopefully forsake the delusive behavior that kept me from facing reality. Dr. Byron, with his poet's name and his direct gaze, might save me from myself. But only if I let him.

159

"Dr. Byron," I forced myself to say, "I am needier than I may appear."

"Mrs. Brownstein," he said with that corn-belt lack of inflection that had been so appealing on the telephone, "we are *all* needier than we appear." Maybe he wasn't Yale after all; maybe he was University of Iowa. Maybe his seedy little foyer was his own ironic stab at his profession. Maybe he was my man after all. I kicked my shoes off and lay back on his couch.

"That may well be true," I said, "but in my case I believe that it is true in the extreme."

"How do you see your case?" he asked so solemnly that when he said "case" it sounded more like "affliction." "What makes you think it's extreme?"

"Forgive me, Doctor," I said, "but I think you've missed the point here. I did not say that I felt my *case* was extreme. What I consider to be extreme . . ." I paused, searching for the words that would clarify my meaning and explain my needs, "what I think is extreme is the *disparity* between how I appear to be taking all that's happened to me, and how I really feel about it."

"How do you think you appear to be behaving?" A good, honest question requiring a good, honest answer.

"Oh, very brave, very strong, very much in control of the ship."

"And that, I take it, is not how you really feel?"

"Of course not," I said. This unburdening was going along much more easily than I would have predicted. "I feel angry and bitter and frightened of the future. And confused and bereft and lonely. Oh God, I feel lonely. And guilty. Yes, guilty, too."

"What is it you feel you're guilty of?" My, I thought, you do jump right in, don't you, mister? About now we were meant to be discussing wigs, not guilt, for crying out loud. This was supposed to be short-term therapy, *very* short term—based on *specifics*. Guilt was not for short-term anything. Guilt was the messy glue of long-term therapy, the stuff that kept you coming to dimly lit rooms like this one for years. Even an innocent like me knew that much.

"Forget guilt," I said emphatically. "That was just an impulse item on my laundry list of emotional complaints. The only thing I feel guilty about is abandoning my family. And I think that's bloody normal. Don't you?"

I had done it. I had managed to break the rules already. In the first five minutes of my fifty-minute hour, I had plunged right into the deep water and asked the psychiatrist to say what he thought.

And still more brazen, what he thought was *normal*. But he was not even rattled. In some strange, inexplicable way it pleased me that he just plodded along, making little scratch marks on his clipboard, and tossing out loaded questions in the cool tone of throwaway lines. In another setting, I thought, Dr. Byron could be a first-rate straight man.

"In what way do you think you are abandoning your family?"

"Do you have children, Dr. Byron? Do you have a family?" I asked. Two could play at Socratic Scrabble®, I had learned in some long-ago classroom.

"Yes, I do," he admitted. "What makes you ask?" I sat up on the couch, crossed my legs and stared directly at him. I could see his eyes now; they were deepset and incorruptible.

"Use your imagination, Doctor. How would you like to be caught in the middle of a storm at sea and see your kids waving from the shore? See them clearly: their eyes, their terrified little eyes. Their tiny fear-clenched fists waving in the distance. How would you like to be hanging onto the side of the boat, praying that you'll make it to shore? Back to those kids of yours?"

"Is that how you see yourself, Mrs. Brownstein? Hanging on?"

"Yes! Yes, that's how I see myself. Hanging on for dear life." He sat back in the wing chair and folded his arms. The clipboard fell to the carpeted floor without a sound.

"Are you afraid to die, Mrs. Brownstein?"

Bingo! I looked at my watch. Only ten minutes had passed since I had come through the door. Dr. Byron looked as though he had just hit a home run with the bases loaded, but I caught his long ball on the fly. End of the scoreless first inning,

"Nope," I said. "I just hate the thought of leaving survivors. Wouldn't you, Dr. Byron?" There. I'd done it again. Your turn, Doc.

"Why did you choose to see me instead of someone who could be available for as long as you might need him?"

Nice dodge of the question, Dr. Byron! He was craftier than I had given him credit for. This was not an Iowa farm boy come to the big city to bring good old common sense to the troubled urban masses. This was practiced, polished. This was professional!

"Why do you keep changing the subject, Dr. Byron?"

"I was not aware that I was changing the subject. You came to me because you wanted to talk about baldness and how to manage that with your children. Isn't that correct, Mrs. Brownstein?"

"I came here, Dr. Byron, for two reasons. One is that I was told you had experience with cases like mine; that you acted as some sort of liaison between patients like myself and Psychiatric Institute. That you were knowledgeable on the subject of brain tumors. I wonder, Doctor: do you ask all of your patients if they are afraid to die or only those you have to cure in a hurry? Before you leave on vacation?"

"Why are you so angry, Mrs. Brownstein?" he said without malice. It was not a question; it was an observation stated as fact.

"Because I don't trust you—any of you. Not your buddy, Melinda Marks. Or Lissal. Or Wong. Or any of you. The truth rang in my head like the Liberty Bell.

"What about Dr. McMurtry? Do you trust him?"

"Yes."

"Why? What makes him different than the rest of us?"

"I like him. Is that a good enough reason? Because if it isn't, there are others. Unlike Melinda Marks, he never frightened me unnecessarily, whereas she seemed to take pleasure in giving it to me right between the eyes."

"For instance?"

"For instance the way in which she handled the preliminary diagnosis. I think she was straightforward to the point of brutality."

"Ah," he sighed. "Perhaps she misjudged you. Perhaps you seemed less "needy," to use your word, Mrs. Brownstein, than you actually were."

"Perhaps, perhaps, perhaps, Dr. Byron. But your attractive female associate has a lousy way with words. And what's more, when it comes to bedside manner, she is not exactly Marcus Welby in drag!" My God, it felt good to say all that.

"And Dr. Lissal? Why do you distrust him?" Pay dirt!

"Because I have read *The Wizard of Oz*. And he's just like the Wizard, an absolute ruler unwilling to show himself."

"You're being oblique, Mrs. Brownstein. Clever, but oblique." I snapped to attention. We were playing with my ball. Shopping for my peace of mind on my dime.

"Okay, Dr. Byron. You want to hear it? Get your clipboard off the floor and hear it all. First of all, I got hit from behind. There were no warnings: no red flags, no sirens, no gathering storm clouds. Nothing. Not the faintest sign of an approaching storm. Not even one wispy little cloud on the horizon. Nothing. *Nada*.

"It came the way the worst storms do—out of nowhere, hitting me full force. Before I even knew what to call it, it had lifted me up and thrown me to the bottom of a black funnel cloud, where it spun me around until I didn't know which way was up. Got that? I didn't know up or down or sideways. But I sat in that dark cloud, and I kept still. Because those were my instructions—my only instructions. Just sit tight like a good little girl and wait. Wait for Dr. Lissal. And while I sat there waiting, that cloud kept spinning me around.

"Do you know what that spinning felt like, Dr. Byron? It felt like the pneumoencephalogram all over again. You know what that is, don't you, Doctor? Sure you do. You can probably hear the screams all the way over in your office at Psychiatric Institute, can't you?" Hot, blistery tears clouded my vision so that I could not see him. He handed me a box of tissues. I blew my nose loud and long as a foghorn. A warning in the storm: more to come, more danger. We're not out of it yet. Look out below.

"And then, Dr. Byron, just when I thought I'd never see home again, the skies turned blue, the air grew still, and I thought the storm was over. In the time between the surgery and the radiation, I believed the storm had passed. But I was wrong, Doctor. It was not the end of the storm; it was the *eye* of the storm.

"The winds picked up. Dogs began to howl. The birds grew silent. But it wasn't the tail of the tornado this time. It was a new kind of storm . . . a tidal wave. But not just one tidal wave, Doctor. Not just one giant wall of death that threatens the entire village, devastates it in an instant, and then recedes into the pages of history.

"Oh no! This tidal wave of mine has magic powers! It repeats itself. Every morning it comes crashing and every afternoon it recedes and lets me have a glimpse of the battered shoreline. And then the next morning it comes again. A solid wall, Dr. Byron: 3.2 minutes of solid wall, cutting me off, leaving me alone. I *cannot* be rescued."

I was panting, gasping for breath. And soaking the tissues he thrust at me.

"And I told you this was about wigs," I said, bitter laughter curbing my sobs. "It's not about wigs, is it?"

He did not answer me. He looked at his watch, took some quick notes, and stretched his legs. Anyone who has spent time in the presence of a therapist knows the signals. But I was a neophyte; I misread them. I thought we were just getting warmed up, just tearing down the ice walls. Wrong; we were finishing. I could hear the outer door to his office click. Another patient had arrived.

Someone else was out there doing battle with the flies, making contact with his own demons. My time was up.

"I'll see you next Monday," Dr. Byron said. "Same time." He escorted me to the door, but hesitated just before opening it.

"By the way," he said nonchalantly, "is that a wig you're wearing?" I reached up and touched the synthetic fibers.

"Yes," I said, dismayed. "Yes. It's a wig. I've been practicing, trying to get used to it before I actually . . ."

"Please take it off," he interrupted. So I did. Right there on his threshold, I pulled the wig off my head. My hair was matted beneath it.

"Where is the shunt?" he asked, studying my head. I reached behind my right ear and touched the small rise under my scalp. For a second, I feared he might ask to touch it, too. But he didn't; he merely stood stolidly at the door waiting for me to put the wig back on. There was no mirror and I was too proud to take one out of my purse. I slapped the wig on my head, tugged it down around my ears, and left.

"He wasn't what I expected," I told Neill that night. "He's either a sicky himself or terribly clever. He got me to cry and tell the truth, and he even managed a sly little peek at my wigless head. I guess he wanted to know if we were talking about present baldness or future baldness."

"Did you discuss wigs at all?" Neill wanted to know.

"No, very little, actually. But we were hot on the subject of other kinds of disguises. He sure saw through the Princess Admirable mask in a hurry."

"Did you tell him about your 'stay sane radio station'?"

"No, we never got around to that, either. I'm telling you, Neill, none of it went as I had expected."

IN FACT, NOTHING WAS GOING ACCORDING TO MY EXPECTATIONS during the following days. I had hoped that once the cobalt treatments began, a slow but steady pace would replace the spinning wheel going nowhere since surgery; but that was not the way it happened. It was slow, all right, waking up and going to the same dark room every day. It was almost unbearably monotonous and wearing, but there was nothing steady about the pace of those bleak days.

One day I was up and the next day down. Two steps forward and one step back. During the middle weeks of my radiation course, that was the pattern of my graceless waltz toward the future.

When my hair began to thin, almost imperceptibly at first, I felt a bewildering sense of relief. The long dark hairs that clung to my brush and lay on the white formica counter were visible proof that something real was being accomplished in that chamber every day. Here at last was a sign that things were getting worse—the perverse corollary being that if they got worse fast enough, they would get better that much sooner.

Four nights later I stood at the same sink, holding a handful of my own hair and grinning with wonder: on the very night I lost most of my hair, I regained a sense of my own vitality—I began to menstruate again for the first time since my surgery! The return of normalcy triumphs over the onset of the unnatural. Given the fact that all of the doctors had advised that the trauma my body had endured might make it many months until I would once again bleed normally, I welcomed that bloody flow as a blessed omen: like my periods, my hair would come back in time. Two steps forward for one step back.

I tried to stay light on my feet. I made a worthy effort to make friends with some of my fellow patients in the waiting room. One morning one of those patients was missing—she had died in the night. Two steps back.

For all of my efforts to see the sunlight in the current landscape of my life, there always seemed to be a dark cloud lurking somewhere on the horizon. Melinda Marks, for example, sounded like a thunderclap the afternoon her phone call interrupted the cheerful little ritual of marking off days on my calendar—the days until August 25, the last day of treatment.

"I'm calling to schedule your L.P.," she announced with her usual breeziness.

"My what?" I asked incredulously.

"Your L.P.," she repeated airily. And then, with consonant-spitting enunciation, "Your lumbar puncture."

Dammit! I could remember vaguely that someone at some time had mentioned this procedure. Whoever it was had even put me on notice that it would come smack dab in the middle of radiation therapy; but like so much other threatening information, my subconscious had been sitting on it. Until this moment, I had managed to forget it. Or perhaps I had remembered it by another name— "spinal tap."

I have always considered the words "spinal tap" to be a classic medical euphemism, suggesting a comradely pat on the fanny when it is actually a long sharp needle in the spine. Whatever it was, according to Dr. Marks I had to have one in order to see if the tumor was seeding in my spine. If tumor cells were present in my spinal fluid (and the L.P. would demonstrate that), there was more radiation coming my way. They would finish frying my brain on schedule and then move the machine to a position over my back. In its simplest terms, that meant more radiation. More treatments. More days with the machine. More postponements of life, a giant step backward. In its most compelling meaning it would signify the spread of the tumor. To me, that meant only one thing: *malignancy*. No one had actually said the word to me. They kept calling it "seeding" and said it in tones that bespoke gardens, not graveyards.

Involuntarily, I began to massage my back. "When do I have to have it?" I asked Melinda Marks.

"Oh, whenever," she said lightly. "But with your moving plans and all, I suspect you'll want to get it over with as soon as possible." She was right. If this turned out to be a two-reel nightmare instead of just a short subject horror film, there were plans that needed to be made. We could not go on paying three rents indefinitely, pretending that "California, Here We Come" was a promise, not just a heartfelt wish.

"Will I have to stay in the hospital for it?" I asked hesitantly. The thought of another night at Neuro made my flesh crawl.

"Well," she said, "you're not supposed to elevate your head after a tap because that can promote some fluid leakage at the tap site and give you one helluva headache afterwards. You ought to lie flat for at least eighteen hours to be on the safe side. But in your case, since you live so close to the hospital, you can just rest in my office for a few hours and then we'll toss you in the back seat of a car and send you home." What a way with words the lady had! The way she put it to me, I found myself opting for one more night at Neuro. That decision speaks volumes about how I viewed the prospect of "one helluva headache."

"I have two pieces of good news," I told Dr. Byron when we met the following week. "My spinal fluid is clean and Adam has graciously accepted a bewigged mommy. My baby steps forward are beginning to feel like leaps of progress."

"I knew about the spinal tap results," he said, surprising me. "Dr. Marks keep me pretty well updated. But tell me about Adam. Has he seen you without hair?" He thumbed through the pages of his calendar. "By now you ought to be almost bald." I was impressed; Dr. Byron was keeping up with the "specifics" of my case.

"You're right," I said, patting the wig I had begun to wear out of necessity only two days earlier. "It's falling out in clumps."

His next question was so predictable I could barely keep a straight face while he asked it. "How do you feel about it?" he asked with a tight smile.

"Not nearly as bad as I had expected to feel," I told him quite honestly. I was not about to explain the comforting connection between losing my hair and regaining my menstrual cycle; I could guess what his rational masculine mind would do with *that* piece of feminine mysticism. Instead I told him that I had accurately predicted Neill's response; although he had not admitted to a closet fetish for bald-headed women, neither had he paled at the sight of me. I slept, made love, and brewed morning coffee wearing colorful, concealing scarves.

161

"Tell me about Adam," Dr. Byron repeated. I settled back against the couch and recounted the incident for him.

"Well," I began, "like most things in my life these days, it didn't happen the way I had expected it to happen."

I had expected the wigs to traumatize my children; instead, Todd hadn't noticed at all, and Adam had walked into my room one afternoon to see my desk littered with rectangular pink boxes.

"What are those?" he asked. "More presents for you?"

Until this moment there had been only two questions to which I had well-rehearsed "wise mother" answers: "Where do babies come from?" and "What happens when someone dies?"

In my maternal daydreams, these cosmic questions had always been posed at a time when I was at my motherly best. The dark mysteries of sex would be illuminated while I baked brownies. Death would be confronted in a warm, soothing bath scene.

Instead the subject of sex had been broached while I was brushing my teeth one morning, and the death discussion was held in a sandbox in Central Park. Ashes to ashes, dust to dust, and sand in the sneakers. So it ought not to have surprised me that the question of wigs reared its metaphorical head at a time when I was caught off guard.

"Those are wigs," I said cautiously. "Not more presents."

"What are they for?" Adam asked, "Halloween?" Ah, my darling innocent child. Halloween, what a perfectly logical explanation. How wonderful it would have been to have said yes. Yes, for Halloween.

"No, Adam, they're for me. Because you know those treatments that I go to the hospital for every morning? The ones that make me kind of tired in the afternoon?" Adam nodded soberly. "Well, those treatments are quite amazing, Adam."

"What do you mean, 'amazing'?" Adam asked. For a six-year-old a word like "amazing" is generally encountered on Saturday morning television. The *amazing* Spider Man. "The *Amazing* Adventures of Robot Roy." Amazing does not come in pink boxes on Mommy's desk.

"Well," I began carefully, "those treatments will make my head well by the time they are all over, by the time we move to California. But the interesting part, Adam, the part that has to do with the wigs, is that the treatments will make my hair . . . well, um . . . the treatments will make my hair look sort of . . . yucky."

"Yucky? You mean like 'gross'?"

"Yeah . . . right. Gross." Adam looked me over, slow and steady as a sailor in a bus depot.

"Your hair looks okay to me," he said.

"*Now* it looks okay. Right. But next week or the week after that, it's going to look yucky. Honestly, Adam, it really will." I believed it—telling it to my child with my stomach churning and my face hot, I believed what I was saying for the first time. Even this morning, my comb had seemed suspiciously clogged with loose hairs. It was going to happen.

"When that happens, Adam, when my hair starts to look yucky, I am going to begin wearing these wigs. When my hair stops looking yucky, I will stop wearing the wigs. Understand?"

"Sure," he said. "Can I see them?"

"Of course," I said. So while my heart fluttered and my hands trembled, I did a one-woman fashion show of hair pieces. Yves Saint-Laurent, Givenchy, and Mary McFadden combined don't get from their fall showings what I got from Adam that July afternoon. Not only did he provide cogent commentary on every style ("that one's too bushy—it makes you look like you're wearing an animal on your head"), he made definite and enthusiastic selections.

"That one!" he commanded when I put on the longest-haired wig of all. "That one is the best, Mom. That one looks just like your real hair."

"Then that's the one I will wear first, Adam." Never mind that it felt like my head was encased in a steel helmet that threatened to crush my skull. (Who would have thought dynel could weigh so much?) Never mind. I would suffer in silence. Mothers are supposed to make sacrifices for their children; if this particular sacrifice was slightly out of the ordinary, so was everything else in my life these days.

"How do you feel about moving?" Dr. Byron asked in one of his more obvious changes in subject.

"Eager. Frightened. It's a pretty mixed bag. The only part that throws me is the fact that no one out there knows anything about this. To them we'll just be the new kids on the block. The new kids who happened to arrive three months late. Big deal."

"Do you think it's a big deal?" Dr. Byron asked.

"Yes. Yes, I think it's a very big deal. We are not going to be your average relocated family, Dr. Byron. Not just another statistic in the saga of mobile American society. We have a history, and no one knows it out there." No Edye to cover the emergencies. No Linda to cope with the contingencies. No Dr. McMurtry to trust. No Michael Margolin to turn to for reassurance.

"I could die in California, Dr. Byron, and no one would even know my name."

"Is that what you think, Mrs. Brownstein? That you're going to die in California? That you won't be cured when you leave New York?"

"I don't think it's *likely* to happen that way, Dr. Byron," I said as a headache began to thump beneath my too-tight wig, "but I think it's possible." He handed me the box of tissues, but I waved them away. "I know the odds on brain tumors, marvelous results notwithstanding. But only a brain stuffed with straw could be oblivious to the possibility of dying in this situation. My brain, as a whole portfolio of close-up pictures will testify, is *not* stuffed with straw."

"I know what your pictures show, Mrs. Brownstein, let me assure you of that. And I think you ought to be a lot more confident. A pinealoma is not going to knock you out of the box."

"Care to put that in writing?" I challenged. Dr. Byron sighed, a very exasperated, unpsychiatric kind of sigh.

"There are no written guarantees, Mrs. Brownstein. Not for you or anyone else. You could move to California and die in an earthquake. You could get hit by a truck when you leave this office . . ."

For this professional wisdom I was paying $1.25 per minute. If I didn't interrupt him fast enough I'd be paying to listen to him chronicle $30 worth of disasters and then my time would be up.

"True, Dr. Byron. But I am not afraid of those things that I cannot control. The treatment of my own brain is something that I do have power over, something I can decide. That's what people are about, doctor. That's where we live. In the act of making a decision, we exercise our brains and our humanity."

"But you *have* made a decision, Mrs. Brownstein. You are having radiation to your brain. That is a decision. If you do not trust that decision, it may be that you don't trust the technology."

He was right. Dead right. I didn't trust that machine for a minute, and for 3.2 minutes a day I considered myself its victim, not its beneficiary.

"You need to trust the technology, Mrs. Brownstein. That is what will save you."

"And what if it doesn't, Dr. Byron?" I said in a frightened

164

whisper. "What if the radiation fails? It happens. People get their heads cooked, they lie on that table for five or six weeks and fry, and *zingo*! Two years later they're back for more. What if that happens to me?"

"The technology, Mrs. Brownstein. Think of the technology. Maybe your husband can help you to appreciate it. If your tumor recurs in two years, there will be laser therapy that may cure you. The tumor didn't grow in your brain overnight; it took its time. More time than it takes for the technology to advance. Trust it. Trust the technology. I'll see you next week."

But these were the days of the unexpected and instead of seven days later, I was back in his office, trembling with self-hate and sobbing with disappointment, just forty-eight hours later. I had taken so many steps backward, I couldn't begin to count them.

One day, just one day out of all of those days of treatment, Neill could not be there. An important business meeting required that he be in Washington that morning.

"Reschedule the appointment," he said. "Make it for the afternoon. I'll be on the two o'clock shuttle flight."

"Don't be silly," I scoffed. "I'm perfectly fine, I can take a taxi. Forget about it."

That morning, that one morning, I missed the treatment. My body shook so violently on the table that even the tape on my head could not keep it from bobbing out of position.

"Take deep breaths, Karen," Pat said. "Just take some deep breaths and try to calm down. You can do it. Come on now, Karen!"

It was no use. My heart was pumping too fast, the air was not reaching my lungs. "Take me off," I begged, "I can't do it."

She bleeped for Dr. Wong, some hospital code message that brought him scampering into the darkened room.

"What is the matter, Mrs. Brownstein?" he asked in that cordial tone which had so unnerved me on the first day. "What is the problem here?"

Pat answered for me while I lay panting on the table: "Her husband isn't here today," she explained *sotto voce*, "she says she can't take the treatment. She's shaking too bad to align the machine."

His voice was a dry command. "Oh, you must have the treatment today, Mrs. Brownstein," he said as he stared down at me imperiously.

In the midst of a full-blown anxiety attack, I ripped the tape

165

from my head and sat upright to defy him and all of the others who had congregated in the dark room to see what the commotion was all about.

"No!" I said through clenched teeth. "Not today, Dr. Wong. I cannot take a treatment today. Let me go home! Tomorrow. Tomorrow I will come back here and I will be your perfect patient again. But today I am going home without a treatment.

"I'm sorry," I said to Pat as I got off the table, "it's not your fault."

I walked numbly to the coatrack, put on my lucky jewelry and my sweater, and left the hospital in a bewildered trance.

I stood on the corner of Broadway and 167th Street and tried to regain control of my wobbly body and frazzled senses. My thoughts flew at each other: I had missed a treatment. The schedule had been thrown off. This day, this one lost day, would mean more postponement, more waiting for it to all be over. What had gone wrong in there? Was it just Neill's absence that had made me come apart, or was it something else? Something more? And what good did it do to stand here in the blazing sun and think about it? I was always thinking about it. The demons were in my body. I could not control them with thought. Not even the ones in my brain responded to thought. My brain, however clever or imaginative, could not save itself. Smart and funny couldn't cut it now.

There was a pay phone on the corner. With my head full of bubbles and my pulse racing I walked to it and called Dr. Byron. There was nothing else left to do.

"Get in a taxi and come down to my office right away," he said sternly. More doctor's orders, more commands.

"Are you sure you can help me," I shouted into the telephone as the traffic roared by and the buses breathed their oily fumes. "Because whatever happens in your office today, Dr. Byron, I have to come back here tomorrow and lie down on that table again."

"What?" he said. "I can't hear you. What did you just say?" A bus screeched to a grinding halt inches from the phone booth.

"I said you better be damn sure you can help me!" I yelled into the telephone. I let the receiver dangle and hailed a cab.

YOU BELIEVE IN AMULETS, DON'T YOU?" DR. BYRON SAID when I was seated on his couch. "Your gold mezuzah, your lucky jewelry, all that stuff you cart to the hospital with you every day. Those are amulets. And your husband, your husband is your most powerful amulet. Isn't he, Mrs. Brownstein?"

Rage boiled in my throat, my hands grew hot. "That," I screamed at the psychiatrist, "is the most obscenely inaccurate statement I have heard from you yet! And if you don't stop calling me 'Mrs. Brownstein' while we're discussing my life or death, who the hell needs you? My name is Karen!"

"I am merely trying to help you trust the machine so that you can go back there and have a treatment tomorrow morning, Karen. I recognize that everybody needs a loved one," he said quietly.

"A loved one!" I shouted. "Is that what you call it, Doctor? Well, let me straighten you out. I'm going to have a treatment tomorrow, and the day after that and the day after that. But not because of anything that you have said or done, don't kid yourself. Because when I'm stretched out on the table tomorrow, you won't be out there watching me on the monitor. Oh no! It won't be *your* loved one getting fried inside that room. You are less than an amulet, Doctor. You're even less than that machine. You're a stranger." I sat back against the cushions, exhausted, the fight gone out of me.

"You're wrong, Mrs. Brownstein," Dr. Byron said quietly. "I do care about you. And that machine you are so afraid of is there to help you, not hurt you. Why can't you believe that? You must learn to trust that machine just as you trust Dr. McMurtry. They are equal partners in saving your life. Make friends with the machine."

167

I did not share with Neill a therapy session in which making friends with high-technology machines had been the central theme. It cut too close to my husband's professional bones. Instead, I called my friend the radiologist that night. She concurred with Dr. Byron.

"He's right on top of it, Karen," she said. "Even as we speak they're experimenting with lasers on a malignant pinealoma at Mass. General. I heard about it three days ago."

Very reassuring. Except for one thing. She had said what no one else had said before now: *malignant pinealoma*. Her up-to-the-minute report on medical technology was intended to bolster my confidence, and to some extent it accomplished its aim. But it also posed the greatest dilemma of that summer, a question that would roll around in my brain for months to come: a year from now, or three years from now when I'm typing a short story or unloading the dishwasher and those drums begin to beat in my head, what am I supposed to do? Reach for the bottle of aspirin, or admit myself to the nearest medical center for laser therapy?

In my next session with Dr. Byron I posed that very question. Riding in a cab to his office, my clothes sticky with August sweat, I phrased and rephrased it. As the breeze came off the river along the West Side Highway, I found myself prettying up the language for him, latching onto words like "overreaction," "denial," and "transference." But when the cab took the exit at 65th Street and met head on with the city's humidity and crosstown traffic, I dropped the buzz words and stripped the question bare.

"How?" I asked in the air-conditioned comfort of his office, "given my medical history, how will I ever be able to walk that fine line between caution and hypochondria? How will I know which headache is from too much California wine and which is the one with real bullets?"

"Judgment," Dr. Byron said quietly. "You will use your *judgment*." My first reaction was to discredit his response as just one more of those universal heavyweights he liked to toss into our sessions. "Judgment," like "guilt" and "fear" and "trust," is one of those words that weighs heavily on your vocal chords, reverberates between your ears, and tosses fitfully about in your brain waiting for interpretation.

"What does that mean?" I begged. "When will I know if my judgment is sound?"

"That" he said, removing his glasses and wiping his brow, "is something you will have to answer for yourself."

I thought about what he had said all the way home. It was rush hour in Manhattan; I had ample time to think.

Judgment. Had I not exercised judgment when I made that very first phone call to Mike Margolin? Or was that merely intuition, a mysterious sense of foreboding that had been born in my dreaming unconscious?

When the decision was made to stay in New York to have the radiation treatments, was that not judgment? I realized now that one of the reasons I had been so mistrustful of radiation was because we had been told by California doctors that whole-head radiation represented the most conservative form of treatment. In California, even if they had waited for the tumor to grow large enough to be identifiable on a CAT scan, they probably would have done circumferential rather than whole-head radiation therapy. All of these terms had just been more words in the medical dictionary until I learned that circumferential radiation probably would not have made me totally bald.

It was something I wanted to announce every morning as I walked through those sliding doors: "You know," I longed to shout to the assembled patients waiting there, "in California you might not have to lose all of your hair. In California they probably play music during treatments. In California I'll bet they have gorgeous murals of redwood forests on the walls. And I'll bet there's no orange Naugahyde®, either. Line up the wagons and follow me, you poor devils! We're headin' West!"

But I hadn't gone West. I had stayed in grim summertime New York City and endured. Was that, I asked myself, because of the advice of my doctors and the soft-sell confidence of a man who loved his work, or was that *judgment*? Perhaps it was both. Maybe good judgment was, in part, recognizing when you lacked the skill or knowledge to reach the best conclusion alone. When you acknowledged that you needed help. What was seeking a psychiatrist's advice if not a call for help? What had forced Neill to pursue answers about the Crazy Lady if not that search for judgment?

By the time the cab had crawled onto the West Side Highway, I had come to a preliminary conclusion: judgment was one part intuition and at least two parts experience. I already had intuition.

169

It was suddenly clear to me that experience and the judgment that followed would take time. I could not summon judgment prepaid; it might take months or even years before I knew which headache remedy was the judicious choice. In the meantime, I had my instincts and the advice of those who knew more than I did.

There were still two weeks of treatments ahead of me.

Perhaps I *could* make friends with that machine in this time. On the face of it, it was not the most alluring piece of equipment I had ever seen, but then when had I really seen it? The lights were always out when I walked into the room and I was too frightened to open my eyes during the treatments, when I might have faced the machine in its illuminated nakedness.

Wait a minute, I thought as we passed the 96th Street exit. I *did* have some experience in this realm. Hadn't I had a brief dialogue with the CAT scanner during my last set of pictures? So what if "sssss-click" was not exactly a warm and wonderful greeting. It was worth a try, wasn't it?

By the time the taxi came abreast of the buildings of Columbia Presbyterian, I had made a decision.

The next morning when our sad little parade—Pat, Neill, and I—entered the darkened room, I turned sharply and asked them both to leave—to go out for a few minutes and leave me alone with the machine. They looked at each other with wary eyes, but there was a proprietary note in my voice that could not be denied.

"Go away and leave me alone with *my* machine," I said to them. They obeyed. To their credit, neither of them made any reference to the cataclysmic events of the preceding day, but it was obvious from the hesitant way in which they backed out of the room that they thought this unscheduled and unchaperoned tête-à-tête between patient and machine was a terrible idea. Perhaps even a dangerous idea.

When I was convinced that they were out of hearing range, I spoke to the machine.

"Good morning," I said to the hulking form. My audible voice bounced off the bare walls of the room while the voice in my head told me I was crazy, reminded me that the psychiatrist's advice—"make friends with the machine"—was not meant to be taken liter-

170

ally. A woman who wakes up one day and discovers herself chatting with machines is merely suspect; but a woman who wakes up one day and *decides* to talk to a machine must be certified bonkers.

"What do you think?" I said as I walked tentatively around the machine, touching it lightly here and there on its shiny surface. "Am I nuts or is there a chance that we can be friends, you and I?" I walked slowly around the big room, my eyes glued to the hospital green floor but sneaking furtive, over-the-shoulder peeks at the machine planted in shadow.

"You're not much of a conversationalist, are you?" I said. "Come on now, relax. Lighten up, big fellah," I advised the machine and, covertly, myself. In California, I had noticed, people say that to each other quite a lot with varying degrees of success. But for my machine, the advice did nothing. I grew desperate; any minute now Pat would come back into the room and end this failing experiment. There was only one thing left to do. It was risky, but by now I felt I had nothing more to lose. I went to the doorway, took a deep breath, and switched on all of the lights.

Although it wasn't the first time I had seen the machine, it was the first time I had forced myself to see it clearly for what it was. And this time was different. This time I was not lying flat on my back like some tearful virgin waiting to be ravaged. This time I stood like the adult human being I was and faced the enemy without flinching.

The enemy, as any combat soldier will tell you, does not appear to be nearly so threatening when the lights go on. My machine, my much maligned, grossly unappreciated machine, did not look threatening at all bathed in 600 watts of electric light. It looked cold and lost, and, centered in that cavernous space, it looked lonely.

I came closer to it, my fear somehow having vanished with the darkness. The machine did not return my smile, but it didn't seem to hulk anymore, either. I walked around the far side of it, and just as I was telling myself that there could be no more than peace between us—never a meaningful relationship—I came to a place on the machine where there was a nameplate. "Eldorado" it said in chrome script.

"Eldorado?" I said to the machine. "Funny, you don't look Spanish!"

Although this may not have been the beginning of a beautiful friendship, it evolved into a very satisfactory dialogue. From that time on, each morning I would wait for the lead door to close, and then I would greet my machine.

"Good morning, Eldorado," I would say to my machine. "Do your stuff, kid." And Eldorado would say "ssss-click." As conversations go, it wasn't the Algonquin Round Table, or even the "Dick Cavett Show"; but in its own way, it was very rewarding.

THE ANGEL ARRIVED VIA THE GEORGE WASHINGTON BRIDGE BUS TERMINAL, full of both inspiration and competence. In place of the customary translucent wings and white silk robe, she wore cutoffs and a T-shirt stenciled "Born to Boogie." But she was an angel nonetheless.

"Debora Spink!" I said to her as she stood in the doorway of my bedroom with her overstuffed suitcase in one hand and Todd and Adam jockeying for position to hold the other. "You are a truly blessed vision. My very own *deus ex machina!*"

Debora blushed strawberry pink. "What's that?" she asked, as she came directly toward the bed and kissed me soundly.

"It's a literary term, Deb. It means a savior that comes from out of left field, just when you think the ballgame is over. I thought my ballgame was about over when you called me last week and said you were coming to California with us. Now that you're here, it all looks like extra innings."

"I'm glad," she said simply. "I think I'll go unpack now and let you rest." Adam was fiddling with the locks on her suitcase.

"Did you bring me something, Debora?" he asked when he could no longer contain the question. He eyed me warily. Asking that question was in the top ten of the "no-no list," right after forgetting to say "please" and "thank you," and talking with a full mouth.

"Adam," I scolded, "please do not ever ask guests if they have brought you a present. How many times do I have to . . ."

"Mommy!" Adam said with exasperation, "Debora's not a guest. She's our . . . she's our Debora!"

Our Debora: for the last two summers, a bright-eyed, gawky teen-ager had ridden a Trailways bus from Greenfield, Massachusetts, to New York City to be a "mother's helper" to the

179

Brownstein family. That job description—mother's helper—became inoperative almost from the first. Debora could do everything the mother in this family could do, and in most cases, she could do it better. Debora could direct puppet shows, barbeque a chicken, soothe a hysterical baby, and fold laundry . . . all at the same time. What was most amazing to me was that she could do all this and more at the ripe old age of fourteen! When I was fourteen, I had exactly two domestic skills: chopping carrots and taking out the garbage. Mostly I had talked on the telephone and read *Peyton Place* with a flashlight. I wasn't even fit to be a mother's helper to my *own* mother, never mind someone else's.

But not Debora. By the time Debora came to us in the summer of 1976, she was a poised and lovely seventeen-year-old who managed to forecast clear weather just by getting off a bus. Her long-distance phone call had been brief and to the point: "Karen? This is Debora. I heard about your trouble. I've discussed it with my parents, and if you'll have me, I would like to move to California with you and help you get settled."

If you'll have me? Did Moses ask the Israelites if they'd allow him to part the Red Sea? Did Christ ask permission before he walked on water? From where I stood, up to my eyeballs in moving boxes and drowning in a sea of domestic as well as medical details, Debora's arrival belonged to that category of miracles. So if while making introductions, Adam proudly said to strangers, "This is my mother, my father, my little brother, and my Debora," who could blame him?

While I went for radiation treatments, Debora walked the children to the library and checked out books on California wildlife. While I spent the afternoons resting, Debora repacked the moving boxes that had been so reluctantly opened when our plans were postponed. Debora, all ninety-five remarkable pounds of her, managed to push open the gates to the future, just as I thought they might close to lock me out.

By the second week in August, my waltz toward the future was not yet graceful, but it was far more sure-footed.

Now there were only nine treatments to go. Thankfully, I had never once been badly nauseated, just somewhat queasy during the early part of the day. Like morning sickness during pregnancy, the symptom was usually gone by noon. Food tasted slightly metallic, but I ate most everything, and even cooked some of it myself. My mother still busied herself in the kitchen, but with less obsession and more attention to counting calories.

"Go home, Mom," I told her one morning when we were enjoying an argument over who would marinate the chicken. "Since you gave up the Sara Lee cheesecakes you're no fun at all! Besides, Debora is here now and most of all, Daddy misses you." She paused with a bottle of wine vinegar in her hand and seemed to consider what I had just said.

My father, who had ignored all of his business commitments through the period of my hospitalization and most of my surgical recovery, had returned to their home in Florida three weeks earlier. It was the longest separation my parents had known since World War II.

"Have a heart, Mother," I said. "How long can he go on living on tunafish sandwiches and the generosity of friends who invite him to dinner? I mean it, Mom, he needs you more than I do."

I think what finally persuaded her was the package my father sent me. It arrived via United Parcel while I was at a treatment.

"There's a box for you on the kitchen table," my mother said knowingly. "You'll never guess who sent it."

She was right. My father never bought gifts; according to him that was my mother's responsibility. She would bake our birthday cakes and he would get the tickets for White Sox Park—that was the personnel plan in our house while my brother and I were growing up. Oh, his name appeared on every birthday, graduation, anniversary, and Mother's Day card ever sent to me from my parents, but the gifts these cards accompanied were inevitably selected by my mother.

What my father *did* do was to write to me when I was away at college or living in another city. His long, philosophical letters full of stoic advice and fatherly affection filled a whole box in my "Karen's miscellaneous—Do Not Touch" collection. But shopping for me, actually entering a store with his daughter in mind, was outside his experience. In all of my life, I could recall only one present that he had chosen for me strictly on his own, and that was when I was sixteen—half a lifetime ago. So despite the fact that the bold, left-handed scrawl on the box that I now opened was definitely his, there was more than a little mystery attached to this unveiling.

I glanced at my mother, whose face was impassive now. "Don't look at me, kid," she said wryly. "I'm as curious as you are." I tore

175

open the plain brown wrapping paper, took the lid off the box, pulled apart the tissue paper, and roared. "I don't believe it!" I howled. "I don't believe he did this!"

The first item in the box was a white T-shirt emblazoned with kelly green letters that admonished YOU GOTTA BELIEVE! Beneath that shirt lay another T-shirt; this one was bright yellow and bore in red an even more direct message than the first: IT'S A GREAT DAY! In case I had not yet gotten the point, there was a third T-shirt. This one, bright blue with emphatic black lettering three inches high, announced to the world: I MADE IT! So much positive thinking contained in one cardboard box left me speechless. My mother laughed until she cried.

"Are you thinking what I'm thinking?" she said, gulping for air.

"I don't know what you're thinking," I said through my tears of laughter, "but I'm thinking of my straitlaced father marching himself into some freaky T-shirt boutique and ordering these babies. Can you picture it? A perfectly circumspect, dapper middle-aged man walking into one of those joints and actually *composing* all of this while some long-haired kid sets it up on the machine. All that's missing from this collection is the one that says YOU GOTTA SWING AT THE PITCHES! I love it! It's the only corny thing Daddy ever did in his whole life, and I love it!"

There was more. Nestled beneath the shirts was a tiny black velvet box.

"Go ahead, Karen, open it," my mother urged. On a bed of white satin lay a delicate pin, a 14K gold oval whose only decoration was two Hebrew letters, the letters for *C'hai*—"life." I turned the pin over in my hand. The inscription on the back was equally straightforward: "You made it. Love, Dad."

I handed the pin to my mother in silence.

"That's your father, Karen. You gotta believe."

"I do believe," I told her. "You can start packing."

———————————
———————————
———————————

Although I spent a lot of time admiring those T-shirts and touching that lovely pin, I refused to actually wear any of those gifts in the days that followed.

"At least try on the T-shirts," Neill said as we undressed for bed one night. "I want to see how they look on you."

176

"Not a chance, friend," I told him, "not until the last day of treatment." On that glorious day, I told Neill happily, I would jog down the halls of the Radiation Department, the purple markings scrubbed from my face, my eyes clear, and my breasts jiggling beneath the blazing red proclamation—IT'S A GREAT DAY!

Neill made no effort to hide his puzzlement. "How does such a smart, funny woman come to be so ridiculously superstitious?" he asked.

"Just spit three times, throw a little salt over your shoulder, and consider it my tragic flaw," I replied.

On the night of August 21, Neill and I sat on our candlelit terrace and watched the black river flowing fourteen floors below us. It was our tenth wedding anniversary. Our children were asleep, our Debora was out for the evening, and inside the apartment our belongings were packed and ready for the moving men.

"No tall ships tonight," I mused as Neill popped the cork on a champagne bottle. "The water is as calm and clear as the air. Look! You can see all the lights of the bridge tonight."

We stood at the railing, silent, cherishing the view. A week from now we'd be Californians, and there were no river views in Palo Alto.

"I'm glad we stayed in New York for the treatments," I said, breaking my reverie. "When we get on that airplane next week we'll be leaving it all behind us. Neuro . . . the Crazy Lady . . . Eldorado . . . all of it will belong to another place and time." Neill sighed, gently pulled me to him and sang softly "A sun-kissed miss said don't be late/That's why I can hardly wait . . ."

"Open up your Golden Gate—California, here we come!" I sang loud enough to wake the neighbors.

We went inside and made giddy, intoxicated love.

Later that night, I locked myself in the bathroom and tried on the I MADE IT! T-shirt. It fit like it was made to order.

"How's your sex life?" Dr. Byron had asked when I called him to cancel the last of my scheduled appointments.

"Quite wonderful," I'd answered. "I doubt there are many bald-headed women who are getting what I'm getting."

"Glad to hear it," he'd said. "And your children? How are they faring?"

"They're fine. Mostly they run around the house barefoot and half naked, practicing for California. Once in a while, though,

177

they dress up in boots and snowsuits. I guess kids have their own separation rituals." He didn't comment.

"And the radiation? How is that going?" he asked matter-of-factly.

"Very well, thank you. That machine is never going to replace a Barbara or an Edye, but now I can think of worse things."

Worse things. One of the ways in which my brain had served me so well was by thinking of worse things. It had allowed me to acquire perspective, and a modicum of precious judgment. What an adaptive little organ had come under fire every morning—even while it burned, it had managed to make music and laughter and sense. The Elizabethans had the right idea with their earth, air, fire, and water. A good brain could stand up to them all. And as for their most quotable spokesman, well, Shakespeare too had been right on the money:

> What a piece of work is Man
> So noble in reason

"It sounds like you're doing fine," Dr. Byron said, sounding so much like my Texas hero, Jim McMurtry, that it made me laugh out loud.

"Damn betcha!" I said.

———————————
———————————
———————————

On August 25, the day of my last treatment, Neill and I carried two huge shopping bags through the first set of lead doors. One was filled with items destined for the children's waiting room. When my therapy had begun I had noticed that particular room was barren except for a blank chalkboard hanging on the wall. The children who were patients in Radiation Therapy had suffered alongside the wretched adult victims with tattered out-of-date magazines the only form of diversion in that joyless setting. No more! We brought books and puzzles and a dozen boxes of crayons and colored chalk. "There is enough blankness here." I told Neill. "A clean slateboard is unthinkable."

The second bag held Pat's gift—a ceramic bird, very much like the hummingbirds on the shirt I had worn to Melinda Marks's office three months before. And there was a bottle of fine wine for Dr. Wong and his staff.

For Eldorado I had no gift, only augmented dialogue. When the door closed on me for the last time I said what I had been saying every morning: "Good morning, Eldorado. Do your stuff." On this day, I added a silent, sincere "Thank you and good-bye."

I didn't jog out of Radiation Therapy, I flew. "Never look back, Karen," Ruth had said. "You are free."

That afternoon Neill and I carried still another shopping bag into Dr. McMurtry's office, where I was to have my farewell examination.

"Well now," he said after the examination, looking out from behind the huge, lacy fern I had taken from the bag and placed on his desk. Moments before I had delivered a cactus flower to Melinda Marks's Wedgwood-blue jungle down the hall.

"How do you feel, Karen?"

"How should I feel?" I asked, blinking back tears.

"Cured," he said in that wonderful drawl. "You should feel *cured.*"

"Please say it again," I whispered, letting the tears fall.

"Gladly," he said, grinning. "I don't get to say it all that often: cured. Cured. Cured."

A healthy brain never stops asking questions; but it also knows when it has the right answer.